TBK Fitness Program

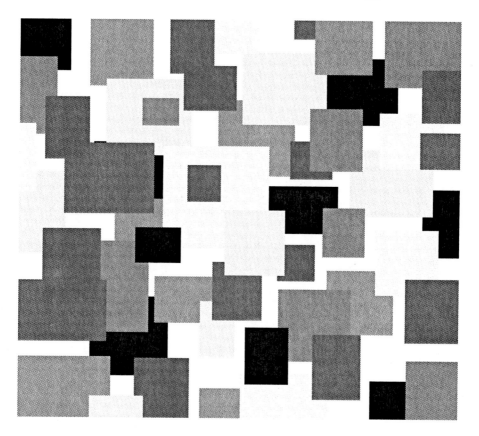

Tamir B. Katz, M.D.

ISBN: 1-4033-9258-7 (e-book)
ISBN: 1-4033-9259-5 (Softcover)

Library of Congress Control Number: 2002095878

This book is printed on acid free paper.

Printed in the United States of America
Bloomington, IN

1stBooks - rev. 03/21/03

Disclaimer:

Before beginning any new diet or exercise program it is strongly advised that you consult with a physician. The information contained in the TBK Fitness Program is NOT intended to replace any diet, exercise routine, advice, or treatment that may have been prescribed by your physician. The author, Tamir B. Katz, is in no way responsible for any physical, mental, emotional, spiritual or financial harm caused by following any part, section, advice, or suggestion found in the TBK Fitness Program. All forms of exercise pose some inherent risk and thus the reader is advised to take full responsibility for his or her own safety, and not to take risks or perform exercises beyond his or her level of fitness, experience, or ability.

Table of Contents

Part 1 – The TBK Diet

Before starting any new diet, it is important to consult with a physician. Although this is a healthy, natural diet, there are certain medical conditions or medications that would make the diet or parts of it unsuitable for you.

Tamir B. Katz, M.D.

Introduction

The basic premise of the TBK Diet is that many of the diseases that plague humanity – such as heart disease, certain cancers, diabetes, obesity, and certain autoimmune disorders result from following an unnatural diet. What do I mean by unnatural? Well, imagine yourself in the woods, or by the ocean or on some fertile plain, with nothing but your own wit. What would you be able to eat? Well, you could gather some berries, fruit, leaves, flowers, roots, nuts, and seeds. You could also use rocks, sharpened sticks, or other simple tools to hunt animals or catch fish. You could prepare simple traps or dig pits and cover them to trap animals, birds, or fish. You might find a bird's nest and feast on some eggs. Water would be the only beverage available. You could start a fire and cook some of the food you have acquired to enhance its flavor, but if you ate it raw you would digest it without a problem, and would still acquire all of the nutrition you need.

You would not have access to many of the foods you are accustomed to today. For example, there would be no dairy products available. You would not be able to catch a deer and milk it. Thus, milk, as well as cheese, yogurt, butter, and cream would not be available.

You would also have little or no access to cereals or grains. Although there may be some wild grains growing around, they would be sparsely distributed, and it would be a waste of your time to gather them and then go through all of the steps needed to make flour out of them. Not to mention your reliance on simple tools, which would make the task even more arduous. Furthermore, there would be no ovens around. Most of your cooking would be limited to roasting over an open fire, making it even more unlikely that you would go through the trouble of using grains to any significant extent. Finally, any grains you would end up eating would be highly unrefined and unprocessed. There is NO way you would be able to make white flour or any other type of refined or processed grains. Most breads, pasta, bagels, muffins, cakes, cookies, crackers, pretzels, and donuts would not be part of you diet at all.

There would be some legumes around, but you would not be able to munch on them raw for any period of time without becoming ill. Instead, you would have to soak and/or cook them to get rid of the numerous toxins and enzyme inhibitors present in order to include them in your diet. However, since you don't have bowls or other containers in which to soak them, and again, since cooking is limited to roasting over an open fire, you probably would not waste your time roasting beans on a stick over a fire. You might come upon some tubers. Most would make you ill if consumed raw, and so, as with the legumes, you would have to soak and/or cook them. Again, any processed tubers would not be included in the diet at all. You would not be feasting on potato chips, instant mashed potatoes, fries, any products containing potato starch, or tapioca pudding.

Sweeteners would be hard to come by. If you were lucky, you could acquire some wild honey. However, you would have to be brave enough to climb a tree with a torch to smoke a bunch of angry bees out of their hive. Honey would therefore be a rare treat. Sugar and other refined sweeteners such as corn syrup and high fructose corn syrup would be practically nonexistent. Thus, once again, all baked goods would not be part of your diet. Neither would candy, ice cream, chocolate, soda and other sweetened beverages.

Alcohol, especially distilled alcohol such as whiskey, vodka, and rum would be unattainable. At most, you might find some fruit that fell on the ground and fermented. But you would not have the equipment to make large amounts of alcohol.

Finally, most oils would in no way be available to you. For example, corn oil. I challenge anyone to produce a drop of oil from an ear of corn without modern machines and chemicals solvents. Soybean oil, cottonseed oil, vegetable oil, peanut oil, safflower oil, sunflower oil, and canola (rape seed) oil would likewise be impossible to obtain. Furthermore, hydrogenated oils, found in margarine and most packaged goods would be unavailable. To produce these harmful oils, one first has to acquire one of the impossible to obtain oils mentioned above, and then heat that oil up at high temperatures in the presence of a metal catalyst. You get the point. Fish liver oil, while potentially obtainable, would become rancid very fast in the absence of refrigeration. You might be able to press some oil out of plump olives, and you could obtain a small amount of coconut oil with some effort. These would be unrefined, unlike most of the oils available in the supermarket, and would be relatively stable. However, even if you obtained these oils, you would probably not be using them for frying, especially deep frying, which requires large vats and a lot of difficult-to-obtain oil.

Human beings who have lived as hunter-gatherers, subsisting on meat, fish, fruit, berries, leaves, roots, nuts, and seeds, and have avoided dairy products, oils, grains and cereals, sweeteners, and most legumes and tubers, seldom, if ever, acquired any of the diseases that are our top killers. However, when these hunter-gatherers become "Westernized" and adopt our unhealthy diets, they develop the same ailments that afflict us. There are two basic questions to ask in order to determine whether a food is optimal for good health:

Would the food in question be available to me if I was stuck out in nature with nothing but a few simple tools (e.g. a sharpened stick, rocks)?

Can I eat the food in question in its raw, unaltered, unprocessed form, extracting the nutrients from it without becoming ill?

If the answer to both of the questions is yes, it is healthy. This does NOT mean that you have to eat the food raw – just that you *could* eat it raw and extract all of the nutrients from it without any ill effects.

However, I advise you to cook all meat, poultry, fish, and eggs because of the potential for bacterial contamination. In nature, if you just slaughtered any healthy animal, bird, or fish, bacterial contamination would not be an issue, and you would be able to eat and properly digest raw meat. However, we get our meat after it has been lying around and handled many times in its journey from the slaughterhouse to our kitchen table, and thus cooking it is important.

Most of us today follow a diet containing a large amount of food which is not readily available in nature, and that must be highly processed to become edible. Our bodies were not made to handle such foods, and thus we suffer by dying of heart attacks, strokes, cancer, and complications from diabetes and osteoporosis.

I am NOT saying that diet is the ONLY cause of the above disorders. Smoking and other tobacco abuse, infectious agents such as viruses, fungi and bacteria, genetic defects, and environmental pollution are well known contributors as well. And obviously, your genes play a role – some people will live to 100 despite smoking cigarettes, while others might suffer a heart attack in their 40s. **What I am saying is that diet contributes a significant amount, and by following a healthy, natural, hunter-gatherer type diet, we can drastically cut down on the number of deaths as well as the significant morbidity (e.g. disability, pain, amputations, blindness) from the aforementioned diseases.** Below, I am going to show you how these unnatural foods contribute to disease, while foods on the hunter-gatherer diet protect one from disease.

Research Studies on Diet and Disease

Before beginning the discussion of diet and disease, I would like to give you an overview of the different types of studies and methods used to obtain data about the different diets and how they relate to disease. I hope the following explanations will enable you to make some sense out of the current nutrition literature, as well as out of any new studies that come out, by judging them based on their strengths and weaknesses, instead of blindly accepting headlines you see in the newspaper.

Each type of study has strengths and weaknesses. At the risk of offending many statisticians, I will greatly simplify the concepts to make them understandable. There are five basic types of studies used to gather information about diets – **animal studies, correlation studies, case-control studies, prospective cohort studies, and intervention studies**.

In **animal studies,** mice, rats, rabbits, dogs, pigs, monkeys, and other animals, some of which are genetically engineered with human genes, are fed different diets. Data is then collected on the effect of these diets on different diseases. For example, a bunch of rats will be fed diet X, Y, or Z. Then, tumors will be induced through a variety of techniques, and the researcher will observe how the different diets protected the rats from tumor growth. Another example is to feed rabbits different diets or foods and then measure how much their arteries clog up from each diet.

At first, animal studies seem to be a good idea. The experiment can be well controlled. All of the rats are housed in the same type of cages, and are fed the same diet except for the specific food being examined. Furthermore, one can control for age, sex, and other traits. Thus, when the results are in, they are most likely due to the effect of the food on the animal's health, and not some other factor. There is an additional advantage of time. Whereas it takes humans years to

7

develop heart disease or colon cancer, interventions can be made to induce such conditions in animals and obtain the data in a shorter amount of time. Finally, whereas it is unethical to try to cause disease in humans, there are fewer ethical issues to worry about when animals are involved. Sounds good, right?

Well, everything's a trade off. There are several disadvantages to animal experiments. They all relate to the fact that ***animals*** are the test subjects, and not human beings. Right off the top, any results obtained have to be interpreted with extreme caution. Unfortunately, this has not always been the case. Rabbits, for example, were fed large amounts of saturated fat, and it was observed that their arteries clogged up after such a diet. From that observation, it was concluded by some that saturated fat clogs the arteries. Of course, rabbits in the wild eat a virtually 100% vegetarian diet, and thus have NO exposure to saturated fats. Thus, applying such an observation to human beings is ridiculous. In fact, many animals, when fed peanut oil (which is low in saturated fat but high in unsaturated fat) develop clogged arteries as well. Animals are vastly different from human beings. Even mammals, or more specifically monkeys, our closest living relatives, are not designed like human beings. They suffer from different diseases, and their bodies react to dissimilar diets differently than our bodies. Furthermore, mice, rats, rabbits, and dogs have relatively short life spans compared to humans. Therefore, you cannot responsibly make diet recommendations to human beings based on the results of an animal experiment.

Another disadvantage pertains to the unrealistic conditions of the experiment. The experiments often consist of feeding the animal a large amount of the study food, much more than even the most gluttonous human being would consume. Also, in most cancer studies on animals the tumors themselves are induced by the researcher to move things along. So, even if a certain food helps to prevent cancer, it might not make much of a difference once you already have cancer. We see then that animal studies are not the best type of study for drawing conclusions about a healthy diet in humans.

The next type of study, the **correlation study,** consists of simply comparing diets and disease rates of different populations or communities, and correlating disease prevalence with dietary components. It is a relatively cheap type of study to conduct, and takes very little time to do. For example, you can compare the diets or specific food intakes of people in the U.S. with that of people in Japan, and then compare the rate of heart disease in the two countries. Or, you could see which food groups are consumed most frequently in countries with the highest rates of colon cancer. Once again, sounds pretty good right?

Well, unfortunately this type of study is probably the most to blame for all of the irresponsible dietary recommendations that we have received, and has probably contributed to the current obesity and diabetes epidemic in the U.S. The problem with drawing conclusions from this type of study is that there could be and often are confounding factors other than the specific dietary component or food that explain the differences in the two populations.

The easiest way to explain this idea is through an example. Let's look back at the differences between the Japanese diet and our diet. Japanese people consume less fat and more soy products than we do. Japanese men also have a much lower rate of prostate cancer than we do. Hence, one might draw the conclusion that if we ate more soy and less fat, we would have lower rates of prostate cancer. In fact, eating less fat and more soy is the message that is being dispensed by the government and most nutritional authorities. However, how do they know that the fat content of our foods and the inclusion of soy in the Japanese diet is what's responsible for the lower rates of cancer? The answer is that they don't know. In fact, there are many other differences between the two populations. Japanese people eat much fewer dairy products than we do (most Asians are lactose intolerant), and there is some evidence that the high calcium intake from drinking too much milk might deplete vitamin D stores in the body, which help protect against prostate cancer. Japanese men are also leaner than we are, a fact that is also relevant since some studies suggest that consumption of too many calories, regardless of their source, might be a risk factor for prostate cancer. Japanese people also have a

9

healthier ratio of n-3 to n-6 fats (which I will discuss at length below) than Americans. Thus, telling the public to eat less fat or eat more soy to decrease their chances of developing prostate cancer might be erroneous.

The nutritional dogma against fat and especially saturated fat began in a similar way. People observed that in certain under-developed countries where people ate less fat and saturated fat, the rates of heart disease were lower than in industrialized countries. That observation, along with some experiments performed on rabbits and monkeys, were largely responsible for the dietary recommendations to eliminate fat from the diet. This has been a disaster for us. We eat less fat today than 30 years ago. However, not only has the incidence of heart disease not decreased despite the fact that a lot fewer people smoke today (smoking is a risk factor for heart disease), but in addition, the rate of obesity, and with it diabetes, has soared since these recommendations were made. The rate of diabetes and obesity has gone up every year since the early 1980s. What went wrong? Well, I'll go into more detail below, but the bottom line is that people replaced fat with processed starches and sugars, which are unhealthy and fattening.

When comparing populations, researchers should be honest and examine the population as a whole. Taking a small part of the Japanese diet and making it a dietary recommendation for Americans is quite frankly irresponsible. Furthermore, although Japanese people have lower rates of heart disease, breast cancer, and prostate cancer, they have much higher rates of stroke, stomach cancer, and esophageal cancer, among others.

The Japanese diet is much higher in sodium, and a higher percentage of Japanese men smoke than do Americans. Thus, living the Japanese lifestyle isn't necessarily the road to optimal health (although I used the Japanese diet as an example, this is in no way intended to put down the Japanese people. I can make the same type of argument with any other population).

The bottom line is that although comparing the diets or dietary components among countries and correlating them with disease prevalence rates can show trends, this is only a starting point that should be further explored before dietary recommendations are made.

The next type of study is the **case-control study.** In this type of study, the diets of a number of people with a certain disease, say breast cancer, are compared with the diets of a number of disease free subjects. The women in both groups are matched as closely as possible for as many factors which might contribute to breast cancer as possible, such as age, family history of breast cancer, weight, use of hormone replacement therapy, smoking status, etc. Presumably, the only difference that remains is the diet or dietary component being studied. One can then mathematically calculate the chance of developing breast cancer with respect to a certain food or food group. For example, 1,000 women with breast cancer are matched up for age, weight, prior history of breast cancer, family history of breast cancer, use of contraception, and alcohol intake with 1,000 cancer free women. Information is obtained about differences in starch intake between the two groups. If the women with cancer consumed on average a much larger amount of starch than the women without cancer, one could make a conclusion that eating starch *may* increase your rate of breast cancer. The case control study is thus a better study than a correlation study because it is better controlled. It is more likely that the dietary variable may be contributing to the disease being studied rather than some other unrelated factor. Another advantage is that relatively rare diseases can be studied. I will elaborate on this point further when discussing prospective cohort studies.

There are still several problems with case-control studies. The first problem is collecting accurate information. People who already have a disease, breast cancer for example, might have an inherent bias when recalling the food that they ate. For example, if the patient believes that eating fat contributed to her breast cancer, she might remember eating more fat than she actually did. Even if there is no bias, recalling past dietary intake is often inaccurate. A second problem lies in the quality of the controls. For example, if all of the cancer patients are matched up with controls who are nuns living a serene life in a convent, some of the differences in cancer rates might be explained by the lack of stress, perhaps better access to medical care or more awareness, etc. A good case-control study will really control for almost every trait so that the results will be more accurate. Even factors such as education level and place of residence can make a difference. Finally, there could be dietary confounding factors, just as is the case with all studies. For example, let's say that women who ate more fat had higher rates of breast cancer. However, if these women also tended to eat fewer fruits and vegetables or more junk food, or if they exercised less, these could be the factors responsible for the higher rate of breast cancer.

Prospective cohort studies, *provided that they are well planned and controlled*, are probably the best type of study to collect information about diet and disease. A prospective cohort study consists of following a large number of people (called a cohort) who are disease free at the onset of the study for many years to decades until they develop the disease, for example heart disease. The end point of the study is when a patient either suffers a heart attack, or dies as a result of one. Through the years, the diets of the study participants are routinely recorded, along with information on blood pressure, smoking status, weight, etc. As you can see, this type of study has many advantages. First of all, the information on diet is collected before the subject develops the heart disease, so that there is less bias about what he or she ate. Second, you don't have to worry about finding controls which match the subjects who developed the disease, since the study population as a whole acts as its own control (i.e. the people in the study who didn't develop heart disease act as the controls for those who did). Third, a wealth of information can be collected on many different diseases, whereas with the case control study, only one particular disease is studied.

The major disadvantages of course are time and money. It costs A LOT of money to track thousands to hundreds of thousands of people for many years. Furthermore, the fact that at the very least you are waiting several years (and often times decades) for enough people to develop heart disease, colon cancer, or diabetes, means that results won't be in for a long while. Another disadvantage is that rare diseases cannot really be studied. For example, say I want to study the potential effect of diet on a rare type of cancer. If only 1 out of 500,000 people develop that cancer every year, it would be impossible to collect enough data, since in your study group of say, 100,000 people, on average, only one case would come along every five years. To get a large enough sample of people to be able to perform a statistical analysis, one would have to wait potentially hundreds of years. That's where a case control study would make more sense, since you find the few hundred or so people who have the rare cancer at present, and match them up with healthy controls instead of waiting for enough disease free people to produce one person with the rare disease. Finally, we have the confounding factor problem once again (the results could be due to a different dietary component or other, non-dietary factor).

The last type of study is the **intervention study.** The usual way an intervention study is set up is that you take a bunch of people with a disease, for example hypertension. You take half the patients, and perform an intervention on them, such as giving them medication and/or a special diet. The other half of the people are either given a fake pill called a placebo, or are allowed to eat a normal diet (or both). The study is done to determine whether the particular intervention is beneficial in either treating the disease, preventing the disease, or preventing complications from it. In our example, the diet or medication would hopefully reduce the blood pressure and prevent stroke and/or kidney disease. An intervention study can take place over many years or can be as short as a few weeks. The benefit to an intervention trial is obvious – if it is successful, it provides a regimen for the successful treatment of hypertension or whatever other disease is being studied.

There are several disadvantages, however, with respect to diet. Most of the time, a healthy diet is only part of the intervention. Often times a medication and or other intervention is added on. For example nowadays, most intervention studies that focus on heart disease include a potent cholesterol-lowering group of medications known as statins in addition to the prescribed diet. Consequently, much, or all of the benefit might come from the medication. Even the studies that don't include medication might use smoking cessation as the additional intervention. Since smoking is a known risk factor for heart disease, quitting may be what's helping the test subjects more than the diet.

If diet is the only intervention, different foods are often lumped together, such that you can't tell which of the foods is responsible for the observed benefits. For example, if you look through the nutrition literature, you will often see a study in which one group of people were put on an unprocessed diet of fruits and vegetables, whole grains, fish, chicken, and low-fat dairy products. The other group eats what they want, which is typically processed grains and starches, sugars, dairy products, processed meat, processed oils and fats, and low amounts of fruits and vegetables. Now gee, which group do you think will fare better? Of course the first one. Here is where things get tricky. Most if not all of the benefits came from eating fresh fruits and vegetables and a small amount of processed food. However, many different conclusions will often times be drawn that are not supported by the evidence. For example, it isn't necessarily true that low-fat dairy products or eating less fat are of any benefit. And of course, whole grains are healthier than processed white flour products. The danger is that the lay public will be preyed upon by misinformation from the food industry.

Few if any of the grains we consume are whole grains. However, any crap that has white flour in it is called grains (the distinction between whole grains and grains is often lost), and people start consuming more of a food that is harmful. Look at the back of any grain product such as crackers, pretzels, etc, and I bet you it will have something stating how it's a grain, and a diet rich in grains can prevent heart disease and certain cancers, or something to that effect. In fact, the opposite is true. The product often contains white flour and hydrogenated oils and sodium which will most likely make you sick, not prevent illness. Another conclusion that is drawn is to eat less fat. Again, the consequences are tragic. People replace fat with processed grain products, and in the long run become obese.

Finally, there are intervention trials which actually harm the patient. Many times, researchers initiate an intervention based on too little evidence, and the result is that more people are hurt rather than helped. In such cases, the trial is often terminated prematurely (since it would be unethical to continue an intervention which one knows is harming the patient).

Before concluding our brief look at the different types of studies used to evaluate diets, there are a few other details to discuss in order to make you understand the various studies. One is how the study was done. For example, many studies use too few people to be able to perform a definitive statistical analysis. This isn't in and of itself a bad thing. Often times scientists simply want to determine if there is a potential trend or interaction between diet and a disease and so they will do a small pilot study to save money (it doesn't make sense to conduct a large, time consuming, expensive study if there is no solid scientific basis to support it). However, conclusions should not be drawn until a further study or group of studies is performed to confirm the results of the pilot study.

There are several other factors to look at, but a detailed analysis of all of them is beyond the scope of this work. One last factor that I want to examine that can affect the integrity and the results of a study is the "conflict of interest" factor. You see, there is a lot more going on behind the scenes than what meets the eye. I don't mean to sound like a conspiracy theorist, but when money or pride is at stake (almost always money), the results of the studies are often affected. Say for example, a multi-billion dollar industry wants to make money off of its product, which has some alleged health benefits. The various companies in that industry would do their utmost to prove that their product actually does work. Therefore, they will fund research studies to prove that it does, and lobby the government or take other measures to suppress evidence that it doesn't, or worse yet, that it is actually harmful. Because so much money is at stake, the results of their own research are often skewed if they don't prove what the company set out to prove. This includes falsifying data, throwing out negative results, and/or playing with the statistics and drawing ludicrous conclusions from poorly conducted studies and using these as the basis for health claims on products. Watch out for this bias and

15

scrutinize every study on any product or food that is supported financially by a party with a monetary stake in the conclusions.

I hope I have given you some helpful tips to wade through the quagmire of research studies on diet and disease, thus enabling you to educate yourselves. Next I'm going to shed a fresh perspective on what foods affect and contribute to disease and what foods help to protect against it. We'll start off with killer #1 for both men and women – heart disease.

Heart Disease

Heart disease is still the biggest health problem we face today, despite long running, expensive efforts to find ways to prevent it. Fewer people *die* from heart attacks today than in the past few decades, but the incidence of heart disease, that is, the number of people who develop heart disease each year, has not decreased. This, despite the fact that fewer people smoke today than in the past. The only reason fewer people die from heart disease today is because of the amazing medical interventions in existence, including bypass surgery, angioplasty, stents, and effective medications.

Eat a low-fat diet. Cut down on saturated fat and cholesterol. Sound familiar? Unless you have been living in a cave for the past 40 years or so, that is the advice you have heard as the way to prevent heart disease (as well as cancer, diabetes, and obesity as we shall see below). However, this advice never panned out. More and more studies today are showing that there is no real link between saturated fat consumption and heart disease. Yes, you read correctly. Saturated fat isn't really it. Neither is cholesterol. The advice that was so simple, wrapped up in a neat little package, turned out to be mostly wishful thinking.

If it isn't fat or saturated fat, then what is it? Furthermore, how did the idea originate that saturated fat leads to heart disease? What roles, if any, do other types of fat have in the causation and prevention of heart disease as well as other diseases? Let's start off with a discussion of the different types of fat, which will help to address these questions.

By now many of you know that there are saturated fats, unsaturated fats, and *trans* fats. Unsaturated fats can be further subdivided into monounsaturated fats and polyunsaturated fats, and two subcategories of polyunsaturated fats are the omega 3 (n-3) and omega 6 (n-6) fatty acids. Those too can be subdivided but to keep

17

things from getting too confusing, we'll stop there. Saturated fats too can be subdivided. Contrary to what most nutritionists tell you, not all saturated fats are the vicious cholesterol-raising villains they are purported to be.

So, where are all these fats found? What is their effect on the human body? What is the difference between a saturated and an unsaturated fat? Well, all fats contain chains of carbons, which are attached to various amounts of hydrogen atoms. If every possible hydrogen that can be bound to the chain of carbons is bound, you have a saturated fat, that is, its carbon chain is saturated with hydrogen atoms. If, on the other hand, two of the carbons are connected via a double bond instead of a single bond, two fewer hydrogen atoms can bind to the carbon chain, and so you get a monounsaturated fat. If the carbon chain has more than one double bond, it is polyunsaturated. We'll get to *trans* fats later.

These different types of fats have different levels of stability. Some of the oxygen molecules we breathe, as well as various other molecules, occasionally lose an electron and become what are known as free radicals. These look to "steal" an electron from another part of the body. As you can probably see, free radicals can cause many problems. Let's say for example, they steal electrons from a DNA molecule or other essential component of our cell. This could lead to cell death or cancer. Luckily, our bodies were created with various defense mechanisms. We have enzymes that repair our cells and DNA, and we produce substances known as antioxidants which neutralize free radicals. Fresh fruits and vegetables contain large amounts of antioxidants as well, which is why it is important to emphasize them in our diets. So what does all this have to do with fats? Well, one of the places where a free radical can steal an electron is from the double bond of a fat. Now the fat is missing an electron and so is going to steal one from another place, subsequently setting off a whole messy process in the body that results in much damage. Well, the more double bonds a fat has, the more prone it is to getting attacked by a free radical. Thus, a saturated fat is the most stable. It has no double bonds, and so free radicals can't touch it. Monounsaturated fats have one double bond, and so are still relatively stable (although not as much as saturated fats). Polyunsaturated fats are the most unstable. They have more than one double bond and so are easy prey for free radicals.

When the fats we eat are digested, they end up in various places in the body, including the cell membrane and the LDL molecule, which transports cholesterol. Many of you know LDL as the "bad cholesterol," but that isn't the whole truth. The LDL in and of itself is harmless. It simply performs an essential function in the body. What happens is that fatty acids in the LDL molecule suffer free radical damage, and this damaged molecule cannot be cleared from the blood by the liver since it isn't recognizable by the liver's receptors anymore. Thus, it floats around aimlessly with its cholesterol cargo until certain immune system cells known as macrophages engulf it along with the cholesterol in it. However, they cannot break it down and become what are known as foam cells, which lodge in the arteries and end up forming clogging cholesterol plaques.

Thus, the more polyunsaturated fats we eat, the more likely an LDL molecule will be damaged and end up contributing to arterial plaque formation. Also, the more LDL molecules we have floating around in the blood, the more likely we'll have plaque formation since a certain percent of LDL molecules will always get damaged. So ideally, we want to consume fats that don't raise our LDL levels, and are stable so that the LDL molecules we do have are less likely to be damaged.

Furthermore, it turns out that there are two types of LDL molecules, subtypes A and B. A are large, "fluffy" LDL molecules, while B are small, dense molecules. It turns out that those with predominantly subtype B LDL molecules have a much higher risk of heart disease. Although genetics play somewhat of a role, the amount and type of fat we eat can affect the proportion of LDL molecules from each subtype.

Finally, we have HDL molecules which pick up cholesterol from the body and transport it back to the liver. The more HDL molecules we have, the less cholesterol that's available to potentially damage our arteries. Thus fats that increase our HDL levels are also beneficial.

So, what fats do what? Let's start off with saturated fats, the most misunderstood of all fats. The carbon chain in the various saturated fats is of different lengths, and that makes a difference in what effects the saturated fat has on the body. Chain lengths of 12 (lauric), 14 (mystiric), and 16 carbons (palmitic) raise both the HDL and LDL levels in the body. They are stable fats because of the lack of double bonds in the carbon chain, and do raise the HDL, or "good" cholesterol; on the other hand they also raise the LDL cholesterol. However, it turns out that saturated fat also shifts the proportion of LDL molecules from the harmful subtype B to the more innocuous subtype A. So even although the LDL is raised, many of these new LDL molecules are of the less harmful variety.

Several decades ago, scientists made the observation that consuming saturated fats increased total cholesterol. Since people with elevated cholesterols were observed to have higher rates of heart disease, it was assumed that eating saturated fats would increase the risk of heart disease. However, this isn't exactly true. Several studies from the past few years have found no increased incidence of heart disease in people who consumed more saturated fat. For example, France, where red meat and dairy fat intake is amongst the highest in Europe, has one of the lowest rates of heart disease. In Spain – where over the last few decades, people have increased their consumption of meat, saturated fat, and total fat (and decreased their intakes of sugars and other carbohydrates) – heart disease and stroke rates have decreased.

It turns out that many of the original saturated fat – heart disease studies compared Western populations who consumed higher levels of saturated fat with populations from poorer countries who ate less saturated fat and had fewer cases of heart disease. However, the inherent fault of these studies is the sheer number of confounding variables. People in Western countries also eat much more processed food, more refined carbohydrates, more sugar, more dairy products, and tend to be fatter and less physically active, all of which may lead to heart disease. The newer studies have done a better job of controlling for many of these variables and it does not look as if it is the saturated fat per say that is contributing to the development of heart disease.

If you think about it, what do most people eat foods which contain saturated fats with? Butter with white bread toast. A hamburger on white bun with french fries and a soda. Steak with potatoes, white dinner roll, and dessert. You get the point. Most of the time, foods which contain saturated fats are consumed with refined, processed starches and sugars. It's these processed carbohydrates that could actually be contributing to heart disease and not the saturated fats. Further down, I'll discuss the mechanism by which highly refined carbohydrates contribute to a whole range of diseases, including heart disease. Interestingly enough, there is a way to measure how much processed carbohydrates a person is eating called the glycemic load, which I'll elaborate on later. If we found a study which controlled for glycemic load, and still found that saturated fat had a substantial effect on heart disease, then we might have more reason to believe the relationship is true. As of this writing, no such study is out there. However, there are studies which controlled for fiber intake, which is a rough inverse correlate to glycemic load (the more fiber in the carbohydrate, the less processed it probably is). And lo and behold, those studies showed that saturated fat barely affected a person's chances of developing heart disease.

Another possible confounding factor which is never controlled for is milk intake. It turns out that milk protein (casein) and milk sugar (lactose) intake has an almost perfect correlation to heart disease. The correlation is much stronger than for any other dietary component, including saturated fat, animal fat, eggs, etc, although the reason behind this observation isn't clear. Although correlation studies aren't the strongest type of study to show causation, such a strong correlation at the very least suggests that something may be going on. Thus, milk intake should be controlled for, especially since much of the saturated fat in Western countries comes from milk and other dairy products.

In addition, several studies, including a decent sized prospective study published in the prestigious Journal of the American Medical Association (JAMA), have shown that people with the *lowest saturated fat* intake have the highest incidence of ischemic stroke (the most common type), although the mechanism isn't clear yet.

A saturated fat with a carbon chain length of 18 is called stearic acid. It is found mostly in beef fat and chocolate. Beef fat contains about 36% monounsaturated fat, 26% palmitic acid, and 21% stearic acid. Stearic acid does NOT raise LDL levels, and one study shows it may even lower them. Furthermore, it does not increase thrombotic risk (a major precipitator of heart attacks and strokes).

Last on the list of saturated fats are the short and medium chain saturated fatty acids, found naturally mainly in coconuts. They do NOT raise LDL levels either, and have various health benefits for the colon, as well as anti-cancer and antiviral properties.

The bottom line on saturated fats is that you should include them in your diet. I am NOT saying to eat them exclusively, balance is important. But, the fact remains that they probably do not contribute much, if anything to the development of heart disease, and avoiding them completely may greatly increase your risk of stroke. Also, don't forget that very few foods are pure saturated fat. Butter for example, is about ½ monounsaturated fat, and as I mentioned above, beef is also only about ½ saturated fat. (only ¼ of which actually affects cholesterol levels). Sadly enough, with all of the advice to reduce saturated fat intake, people have been replacing beneficial foods such as fresh meat and its plethora of nutrients with processed carbohydrates, and thus we have the current obesity and diabetes epidemics in this country. The current thinking is often "A bunch of fat free cookies with a large soda are fine, but I will not touch that steak with a ten foot pole."

Next I will discuss the n-6 fatty acids, which are a subgroup of the polyunsaturated fats. These are, aside from *trans* fatty acids, the worst group of fats to consume. We do require a small amount of them for daily body functions, but we consume much higher amounts than we should, to the detriment of our health. Although they lower LDL cholesterol levels, they also reduce HDL levels, and because they have several double bonds, they are very prone to attack by free radicals. These attacks lead to higher levels of damaged LDL molecules, which, as stated above can lead to clogged arteries. N-6 fats also induce an inflammatory environment in the endothelial cells of our arteries, which can also promote clogged arteries. Studies have shown that they may also contribute to high blood pressure. Furthermore, several studies suggest that n-6 fats may be carcinogenic, promoting tumor growth and formation of new tumors. It gets worse. It turns out that n-6 fatty acids are converted into substances that promote inflammation in the body by overexciting the immune system. These substances exacerbate such conditions as rheumatoid arthritis, asthma, chronic obstructive pulmonary disorder, ulcerative colitis, psoriasis, and allergies, amongst other things.

Think that's it? Nope. N-6 fatty acids may also fatten you and cause insulin resistance, a condition that leads to diabetes. Americans eat more n-6 fats than almost anyone in the world, and it shows. We are probably the fattest nation on earth. The sad thing is, many nutrition "experts" recommend these n-6 fats as "heart healthy" fats because of the superficial observation that they reduce LDL levels. These damaging fats are found in large amounts in virtually all vegetable and seed oils with the exception of olive oil, flaxseed oil, and coconut oil. These include soybean, corn, canola, cottonseed, sunflower, safflower, peanut, and sesame oils. They are also found in mayonnaise made from the above oils, and in smaller amounts in chicken, pork, and somewhat in beef fat, as well as most other foods that contain fat.

At this juncture, I would like to address an important point regarding animal fats. Bear with me and you'll see the relevance to the current topic. One of the reasons that animal fat tends to be unhealthy is that in this country, and in most of the industrialized world, animals are force-fed unnatural diets. They are fattened with grains, corn, and soybeans, and so the fatty acid content in their bodies tends to be higher in n-6 fatty acids. Furthermore, they are force-fed and fattened with high carbohydrate diets, leading to high amounts of unnatural intramuscle fat (It is ironic that the same foods that farmers use to fatten their animals are promoted as healthy by the government and many leading nutritionists. Perhaps this also explains why we as a society are so fat and unhealthy). This is also true for eggs from grain fed chickens. They contain more n-6 fatty acids than eggs of chicken in some other countries where the chickens are allowed to graze and eat a partially natural diet. Wild animals eat mostly leaves and grasses, not seeds or grains. It turns out that leaves and grasses contain beneficial n-3 fatty acids (see below) while grains and seeds are higher in n-6 fatty acids, and thus the fatty acid profiles of wild animals are better than those of their domestic cousins.

In conclusion, I advise all of you, whether or not you follow the TBK diet or not, to stay away from foods containing large amounts of n-6 fats, and to choose leaner cuts of meat and poultry, since their fatty acid content has been worsened by force feeding them an unnatural diet. If you can afford it, game meat such as venison and bison and n-3 enriched eggs are a smart investment.

On to n-6's benevolent cousin, n-3. These fatty acids pretty much have the opposite effect as n-6 fats in virtually every situation. They lower the risk of clots and arterial inflammation, which may reduce the risk of heart attacks. Although some studies show that n-3 consumption may not necessarily reduce the incidence of heart attacks, it lowers the risk of sudden death from cardiac arrhythmias by insulating and stabilizing the heart cells from aberrant electrical impulses that can lead to the fatal arrhythmias. These fatty acids are converted in the body into substances which lower blood pressure and prevent inflammation and the inflammatory diseases listed above. Studies have shown n-3 fatty acids also lower the risk of cancer, and may inhibit the growth, spreading, and formation of tumors. They are found mainly in fish and seafood, but also in flaxseeds and green leafy vegetables, as well as the meat of wild animals, which eat green leaves rather than grains and soybeans. These are among the best fats to emphasize in your diet. Some studies have suggested that people who eat more fatty fish tend to be healthier. Eskimos, whose diet is mostly seafood, have almost no cases of heart disease.

A hunter-gatherer type diet such as the TBK diet contains a natural ratio of n-6 to n-3 of less than 4 to 1, while in the typical Western diet, this ratio is more like 14-20 to 1. This too might explain our high disease rates. Most packaged food in the Western diet is devoid of any n-3. It contains either n-6 fats or the more harmful *trans* fats, to be discussed below. Furthermore, grains and legumes also contain much more n-6 than n-3 fats. The typical diet followed by hunter-gatherers living in the wild is rich in leafy vegetables, fish, and wild game meat. The only sources of n-6 fats are walnuts, brazil nuts, and seeds which if eaten in moderation, do not constitute a problem (after all, how many of you sit there eating entire bags of walnuts or brazil nuts).

There are those of you who might be wondering why n-3 fatty acids aren't also damaged by free radicals since they too are polyunsaturated. Well, they are. But, there are several reasons why you don't have to worry about it. First of all, even foods that contain high levels of n-3, like fatty fish, only contain a few grams at most per serving. Second, the benefits of n-3 fatty acids through their protective effects on the body far outweigh the potential free radical damage they receive in the body when taking in account how little of these fats one actually consumes. Third, in the presence of low dietary n-6 fat intake, and with a high intake of antioxidants from fresh vegetables and fruit, the amount of free radical damage is minimal. **One warning I do have is to get your n-3 fats from fresh foods.** Do not go buying fish oil, which can become rancid fast, and make sure your fish is not spoiled (it will smell badly if it is).

In conclusion, increase your intake of n-3 fats, but get them from fresh food rather than oils. These fats have many good effects on the body including protection from cancer, heart disease, inflammatory diseases, and sudden death.

Onto the monounsaturated fats. These include olive oil, avocados, and most nuts (including pecans, hazelnuts, macadamia nut almonds, pistachios, and acorns – walnuts and brazil nuts are exceptions I can think of off hand which are higher in polyun of fats). A lot of nutritionists will try to sell off canola oil as monounsaturated fat as well, but I don't buy it. Although it does have a fair amount of monounsaturated fat in it, it also has a relatively large amount of n-6 fat and so I don't recommend its use. Olive oil is relatively stable and resistant to free radical damage. Furthermore, since monounsaturated fats in general tend to raise the good HDL cholesterol, while lowering the LDL cholesterol, olive oil is one of the best fats to eat. I use olive oil exclusively. If you can take the flavor, buy extra virgin grade oil since it is the least processed and contains antioxidants and other beneficial substances. The lower grade oils, especially "light" olive oil, tend to be more processed and if possible should be used secondary to extra virgin oil.

In conclusion, monounsaturated fats are among the healthiest to consume and you should devote a large chunk of your fat intake to these. If you are on the TBK Diet, this shouldn't be hard to do, as you can select from many different nuts (which have been shown by multiple studies to be good for the heart and even for longevity), as well as avocados, olives, olive oil and meat and poultry.

Finally, we come to *trans* fatty acids. I have nothing good to say about these. They have NO redeeming qualities. If you eat packaged foods that have fat in them, such as crackers, donuts, cookies, cakes, popcorn, chips, pies or even breads, chances are they contain *trans* fats. Look at the label. If you see the words hydrogenated oil, or partially hydrogenated oil, you are consuming these horrible fats. What exactly are *trans* fats? Well, when companies want a fat that is liquid at room temperature to be more solid, they hydrogenate it, meaning they add hydrogen molecules to it through a chemical reaction to make it more saturated (and thus more solid at room temperature). The problem lies with the fact that in nature, the double bonds in a fat are arranged in a certain conformation known as the *cis* conformation. Hydrogenating the fats arranges much of the fat in a *trans* conformation, which is rarely found in nature. These unnatural fats find their way into your cell membrane and a host of other fatty components in your body, disrupting them and creating the potential ʳ great harm. Although these fats haven't been studied for a long ˙ and not much is known about them, it is known that they lower ꞏd HDL cholesterol and raise the LDL cholesterol levels. They also promote calcium influx into the arterial cells which can lead to clogged arteries. My theory is that in time it will be found that these fats are carcinogenic and lead to a number of other disorders as well.

It is ironic that the witch hunt against saturated fats has led to the widespread use of *trans* fats. People were told to eat margarine instead of butter with the mentality that margarine was heart healthy. How wrong these "experts" were, at the detriment of our health. The food companies are happy. The hydrogenated fats come from cheap vegetable oils, saving them money, and of this writing, food companies are still not legally obligated to report how much *trans* fats their food products contain. Thus millions of Americans are unsuspectingly damaging their health by consuming large amounts of these fats in all of the baked goods, junk food, frozen meals, and other processed food currently out on the market.

Well, we've come to the end of our discussion of fats. As you will see later on, following a hunter-gatherer diet such as the TBK Diet will give you an ideal proportion of n-3 fats, monounsaturated fats and saturated fats with very little unhealthy n-6 fats, and virtually no *trans* fats.

Before moving on, I will briefly touch on the subject of cholesterol. Scientists in the past observed that the deposits clogging our arteries are extremely rich in cholesterol, and thus assumed that intake of cholesterol might lead to heart disease. However, studies have shown that dietary cholesterol does not significantly increase blood cholesterol levels. In fact, the human body produces about 1 gram of cholesterol on its own each day anyway, and adjusts its own production based on dietary intake. Thus, if one consumes extra cholesterol (by having a couple of eggs for breakfast for example) the liver, which manufactures cholesterol, will produce less that day.

Let's get back to the topic of heart disease. What happened in this country, as I mentioned above, was that people began eating less fat, especially saturated fat. Well, the void left had to be replaced by something else. Since many protein rich foods also contain fat, these calories were replaced mostly by starchy, processed carbohydrates. Nutritionists recommended that we eat more "complex" carbohydrates, namely breads, pasta, rice, and potatoes. And so began the fattening of our country. Not all carbohydrates are harmful. However, the ones that are consumed in the highest amounts by Americans are indeed damaging to the body.

How can you tell if a carbohydrate rich food is harmful or not? It used to be thought that complex carbohydrates, which come from starchy foods, are better than simple carbohydrates. However, the distinction between the two is meaningless. All carbohydrates we consume are broken down into glucose in our bodies. They get broken down at different rates, and this is what is important. For example, a potato, which is a complex carbohydrate, is broken down into glucose much faster than an apple, which contains simple carbohydrates. When a carbohydrate is broken down into glucose, that glucose enters our bloodstream. The body senses the rise in blood glucose, and our pancreas secretes the hormone insulin. Insulin has many functions. It helps the glucose from our cells enter the liver, muscle cells, and fat cells. It also initiates the production of insulin like growth factors (IGFs), which have anabolic properties, promoting growth in the body. Insulin also **shuts down fat burning pathways** and the pathways that use protein for energy (gluconeogenesis). **It promotes fat storage**, and **induces the production of triglycerides** (fat molecules in the blood).

The faster the carbohydrate enters the bloodstream as glucose, the more insulin is required to deal with that glucose. Herein lies the problem. Since insulin blocks fat burning, promotes fat storage, and increases production of triglycerides, which are a risk marker for heart disease, too much insulin leads to health problems. The speed at which a carbohydrate enters the blood stream as glucose is known as its glycemic index. Foods with no carbohydrates in them such as steak, eggs, fish, etc. don't induce much insulin secretion when consumed. Fruits, vegetables, nuts, and legumes for the most part have low glycemic indexes. That is, when you eat an orange or some almonds, it takes a long time for the carbohydrates in them to be broken down into glucose. On the other hand, most grains, sugars and tubers, including candy, bagels, breads, potatoes, rice, and of course all refined grains such as breakfast cereals, many baked goods, crackers, pretzels, and other white flour products have higher glycemic index values. Many factors affect glycemic index, amongst them the actual form of carbohydrate found in the food, its fiber content, and its fat content, the latter two decreasing a food's glycemic index. Fiber is indigestible, and so prolongs the time it takes for the carbohydrate in the digestive tract to become digested. Fat slows down digestion, and therefore the carbohydrate takes a longer time to be broken down into glucose and enter the blood.

The glycemic index isn't the only thing that counts. For example, if you ate a tiny piece of candy, although the sugar in that candy may be digested rapidly and therefore have a high glycemic index, a small piece of candy contains very little sugar, and so it would not induce much insulin secretion. On the other hand, some pastas have glycemic index values which are not too high. However, because they are so loaded in carbohydrates, even if those carbohydrates are digested more slowly, there are so many of them that a large amount of insulin is required. Therefore, we use what's called the glycemic load, which is defined as the glycemic index of a food, multiplied by the amount of available carbohydrates per serving of that food. **Several new studies have linked high carbohydrate diets, particularly those with high glycemic loads to heart disease, as well as certain cancers, diabetes, and obesity**. The foods with the highest glycemic loads are the starches such as pasta, rice, bagels, and potatoes. Of course, the highly refined versions of those foods (e.g. white flour products), as well as heavily sweetened food, carry an even greater glycemic load. Legumes have an average glycemic load, and most fruits, all vegetables, and all nuts have a very low glycemic load. However, some dried fruits, especially dates, figs, and raisins, have a quite high glycemic load. Bananas are also a bit on the high side. Dairy products for the most part have low glyemic loads, but I don't recommend them for other reasons which will be discussed further on.

Replacing fat in the diet with carbohydrates, more specifically those carbohydrates with a high glycemic load, produces a number of harmful changes. As I mentioned above, the high insulin levels cause fat deposition, block fat burning, and raise triglyceride levels. Although total cholesterol levels tend to fall, **HDL levels drop as**

well, and LDL levels shift to the harmful subtype B. In fact, the cluster of high insulin levels, low HDL levels, high triglyceride levels, and a high proportion of LDL subtype B puts a person at a very high risk for heart disease. High glucose levels by themselves also cause damage in the body. Glucose is "sticky" in the blood, binding to many proteins and other molecules in the blood, leading in fact to premature aging. For example, glucose can bind to LDL molecules, rendering them unrecognizable and leading to the same sequence of events as the free radical damage to the LDL molecule described above.

As an aside, this might be one of the reasons that *too much* saturated fat is not a good idea for many Americans who follow a high processed food diet. The LDL levels can increase after increased intake of certain saturated fats, and the glucose levels produced from eating refined foods can glycate those excess LDL molecules. By contrast, eating a large amount of saturated fat in the absence of foods with high glycemic loads is probably innocuous.

The complications of type 2 diabetes (the most common type of the disease), which is characterized by high insulin and blood glucose levels, include damage to most of the blood vessels and many of the nerves in the body, leading to heart disease, blindness, kidney disease, susceptibility to infections, limb pain, and amputations. **The bottom line is that the human body does not deal well with high levels of insulin and glucose.** Of note, the human body has only one hormone, insulin, to lower glucose levels, but four hormones (glucagon, growth hormone, epinephrine, and norepinephrine) to raise blood glucose levels. This reinforces how unnatural high glycemic load diets are, and how unprepared our bodies are for dealing with chronically elevated levels of glucose.

Another marker for heart disease which researchers have noted is homocysteine, a substance produced in the body during protein metabolism. It has been shown that high levels of homocysteine predispose people to heart disease, although the mechanism is not clear. What is clear, however, is that lowering the homocysteine level reduces the risk for heart disease. The most effective method to date of accomplishing this is through supplementation of vitamin B12, vitamin B6, and folate. All three are found in generous proportions in fresh red meat. Thus, we have more proof against the idea that red meat can lead to heart disease. Folate is found in green leafy vegetables and some fruit as well.

Finally, several studies have shown that unfiltered coffee also raises cholesterol levels (mostly the LDL) because of a certain oil in the coffee beans, which apparently stays in the coffee if it isn't filtered. Therefore, frequent consumption of unfiltered coffee should be avoided.

In conclusion, a high processed carbohydrate diet, combined with all of the *trans* fats that go hand in hand with those foods that contain refined carbohydrates, are a deadly one two blow to our health. However, it is simple to avoid this damage. As long as you shun processed food, and stick with fresh meat, fish, fresh fruits, vegetables, and nuts, your insulin, glucose, homocysteine, and triglyceride levels will be low, your HDL high (especially if you exercise), and your LDL levels low and with a higher proportion of subtype A molecules, all decreasing your chances of developing heart disease, and, as we shall see below, several other diseases.

Diabetes

There are two types of diabetes, Type 1 and Type 2. Type 1 is found predominantly in children and adolescents and results from an autoimmune reaction against the insulin producing cells of the pancreas. The patient eventually makes too little or no insulin, and has to be given insulin injections to replace what his or her body no longer produces. Only about 10% of the cases of diabetes are type 1.

Type 2 diabetes, which accounts for approximately 90% of all cases of diabetes, has a somewhat different etiology. It is found usually in overweight, middle aged men and women who also tend to have the cluster of findings I discussed above of low HDL levels, high plasma triglycerides, high insulin levels, and a predominance of subtype B LDL molecules. Thus, the type of person at risk for diabetes is also at risk for heart disease. No one is a hundred percent sure how the disease develops, but there is strong evidence that eating a high glycemic load diet is a strong risk factor, as is consumption of *trans* fats (although this may be a confounding variable, since these fats are often found in foods with high glycemic loads). On the other hand, a large prospective cohort study showed no connection between saturated or total fat intake in the development of diabetes. Once again, it seems as though the advice to eliminate saturated fat from the diet has resulted in poorer health, as people replace fat and saturated fat with processed, refined foods that have a high glycemic load.

The development of type 2 diabetes is thought to occur in the following way: A person chronically, over many years, consumes a diet with a high glycemic load. For years then, the body has to produce high amounts of insulin to cope with such a diet. The person usually becomes obese during that time from the high insulin levels as well as the high amount of calories usually found in foods with a high glycemic load. The high amounts of insulin lead to insulin resistance, that is, the insulin receptors on the different cells in the body which accept glucose, become less likely to recognize the insulin. Thus, in order to effectively get the glucose out of the blood, the body must now produce higher levels of insulin. This of course leads to more insulin resistance. At some point, the body simply cannot keep up with the higher demands for insulin, and so the blood glucose levels rise and the person develops diabetes. In type 2 diabetes, the pancreas may also burn out after being overworked for so many years, further exacerbating the situation.

Unfortunately, diabetes can be around with no symptoms for many years. In fact, people are often diagnosed with diabetes after coming in complaining of a side effect of the disease, such as blurry vision or tingling in their feet. By then, the diabetes has been around for a while and has caused much damage. There is a strong genetic component to diabetes, meaning that many people are much more susceptible to the harmful effects of a bad diet. In some Native American populations, upon adopting Western diets and abandoning their minimally processed ancestral diets, up to 50% of adults become diabetic. Today we are seeing type 2 diabetes in adolescents as well. Just 10 years ago it was extremely uncommon for a pediatrician to ever see a case of type 2 diabetes. Today, unfortunately, more and more of our children are obese and thus more prone to developing diabetes at a younger age.

Once again, the bottom line to avoiding type 2 diabetes is to eat an unprocessed, low glycemic load diet which is also low in *trans* fats, and high in fresh fruits and vegetables, nuts, fresh meat and fish (We are beginning to see a pattern here).

Cancer

Cancer is a whole range of diseases with many different etiologies. It is not known what causes many types of cancer. However, there are several types of cancer which do appear to have a dietary connection including colon cancer, breast cancer, and prostate cancer. Breast cancer and prostate cancer are the second biggest killers and the most common cancer in women and men respectively in the United States (lung cancer is the number one cause of cancer deaths and is largely caused by smoking). Colon cancer is the third most frequent killer as well as third most common cancer in both men and women. Thus we see that a proper diet, along with the avoidance of smoking, can make a HUGE difference in disease prevention.

We'll start off with colon cancer. You may have heard once again that saturated fat, or fat in general, and red meat all contribute to the development of colon cancer, and that increasing dietary fiber intake helps to prevent it. Let's examine the evidence. The vast majority of studies from the past decade or so have shown NO association between total fat or saturated fat and incidence of colon cancer. There is evidence from several studies however that a diet high in starches such as pasta and rice are a strong risk factor for colon cancer. This makes sense, since the high insulin levels that result from such a diet may induce the growth of tumors through various mechanisms such as the IGF release and the direct growth promoting effects of high levels of glucose and triglycerides.

In fact, diabetics, who have high levels of insulin, glucose, and triglycerides, seem to be at higher risk for the development of colon cancer. There is no evidence that fiber protects against colon cancer. However, some studies suggest that an intake of fresh vegetables, in particular onions and garlic, may have protective effects. Some studies have shown that a link exists between egg consumption and colon cancer, but the mechanism is not clear, and the possibility of confounding variables is quite high, since eggs are typically eaten fried, and /or with starchy foods, which, as I stated above, are risk factors for colon cancer. Consuming too many calories and being obese, both conditions related to high glycemic load diets, may be risk factors as well, although the association is somewhat weaker.

The majority of studies have not shown a connection between *fresh* red meat intake and risk of colon cancer. Several have shown a weak connection between processed meat intake and colon cancer. One large prospective study did show an increased risk of colon cancer with fresh red meat intake. However, upon closer inspection, there were possible confounding variables. Although fiber intake was controlled for, as were intakes of several vitamins and several other factors, glycemic load was not controlled for. In light of the fact that a starch heavy diet (which is roughly equivalent to a diet with a high glycemic load) is a risk factor for colon cancer, and the fact that people who eat meat may also be eating potatoes, rolls, or other starchy foods, or may be eating the meat as a pot pie, it would have been worthwhile to control for it.

Furthermore, no biological mechanism has ever been found to help explain any possible connection between red meat and cancer. For example, for a while people thought that heterocyclic amines (HCA's), carcinogenic compounds produced when meat is charred, might contribute to colon cancer formation. However, most studies have not shown any connection except at the very highest levels of intake, which are not applicable in most human diets. Furthermore, HCA type mutations were not found in most colonic tumors, and lastly, HCA's are also produced when fish and poultry are charred, but no connection has been shown between intake of fish or poultry and colon cancer. The high iron content of meat has also been proposed as a possible mechanism, but this too has not been proven. Anyway, it is relatively easy to rid the body of excess iron by donating blood, which I will discuss in part 4 of the TBK Fitness Program.

Finally, a study which pooled data from five large prospective cohort studies showed no difference in deaths from colon cancer between vegetarians and non-vegetarians, which strengthens the argument that it is not red meat per say, but the junk food often eaten with it that probably contributes to colon cancer.

The bottom line is that eating a low starch, low processed red meat, high fresh vegetable diet may protect against colon cancer. Fat doesn't really play a role either way, and fresh red meat doesn't seem to be a factor.

On to breast cancer. Once again, total fat and saturated fat, as well as most other groups of fat have not shown to increase a woman's risk of developing breast cancer. In fact, some studies show that eating more fat at the expense of carbohydrates might decrease a woman's chances of developing breast cancer. However, this isn't true for all fats. There is some evidence that n-6 fatty acids may *increase* the risk of developing breast cancer, and when a woman develops breast cancer, these fats may speed up the growth of the tumor. Starches have been shown to be a risk factor for breast cancer as well, as is obesity. Fiber may have a protective effect, but it is just as likely that fiber is a marker for a diet which is lower in starches and other refined carbohydrates, and higher in fruits and vegetables. Finally, for those of you wondering if red meat is a risk factor, a large study which looked at data from eight prospective cohort studies found no association between intake of red meat and breast cancer.

The bottom line is that, once again, eating a low starch diet, following a more natural, less processed diet and staying lean may protect against breast cancer.

Next we'll examine the evidence on prostate cancer and diet. It has long been observed that in countries where hardly any dairy is consumed, prostate cancer is relatively rare. A recent, large prospective study indeed found an association between dairy intake and prostate cancer. Various factors were controlled for, such as dairy fat (to make sure that it wasn't the fat that is responsible). They found that skim milk intake had the highest association with prostate cancer. The researchers speculate that high calcium intake may suppress the body's production of the most active form of vitamin D, which may protect against certain cancers.

Certain substances in fruits and vegetables (e.g. lycopene from cooked tomato products) may offer protection. As of this writing, no studies have been completed on glycemic load and prostate cancer, but there is evidence that consumption of too many calories, which in this country usually translates to refined starches and fats, is a risk factor. Indeed, IGF and thus insulin plays a major role in the growth of prostate tumors, further lending support to the idea that a high glycemic load is a risk factor. Finally, although some older correlation studies have linked red meat consumption to prostate cancer, a large prospective study, which was better controlled for other dietary components, found no association. Processed meat, on the other hand, was linked to an increased risk of metastatic prostate cancer (cancer that has spread).

The bottom line is that by avoiding dairy products, in particular milk, yogurt, and cheese, and by otherwise following a diet that does not have too many calories, such as the TBK Diet, you can reduce your chances of developing prostate cancer.

Finally, I'll touch upon the risk factors for development of stomach cancer. It seems that once again, a high starch diet is a risk factor, as are salty foods and fermented foods. Smoking and alcohol consumption were also found to be risk factors. A high vegetable intake is protective.

Let's step back for a moment and look at the big picture. In all of the cancers we looked at, eating a diet rich in starches, which is roughly equivalent to a diet with a high glycemic load, is a risk factor. A Swedish team recently made an interesting discovery which adds further strength to the findings that starchy carbohydrates can lead to cancer, even without taking into account their high glycemic load. They found that prolonged cooking of carbohydrates and/or cooking at high temperatures (e.g. deep frying, baking) leads to the formation of a carcinogen known as acrylamide. The highest concentrations were found in potato chips, french fries, crackers, and cookies, but high amounts were also found in corn chips, breakfast cereals, other fried foods and in breads.

Fresh vegetable consumption seems to have a protective effect. Fat doesn't seem to play much of a role, although n-6 fats may have a role in the growth promotion of existing tumors. Smoking, although not technically related to diet, is worth mentioning since it is a known risk factor for many types of cancer, including cancer of the lung, throat, esophagus, stomach, pancreas, colon, and cervix.

Obesity

In light of the current obesity epidemic, I thought it would be prudent to discuss obesity, which many scientists today are calling a bigger threat to our health than even smoking. Roughly 65% of Americans are overweight. Obesity puts both men and women at risk for heart disease, heart failure, certain cancers, diabetes, and joint problems. The epidemic is largely due to misguided dietary recommendations by the government and nutrition experts coupled with the abundance of processed, high calorie junk foods.

Originally, the experts gave us the same advice for reducing our waistlines as for reducing the risk of heart disease, namely, to cut down on the fat in our diet. The logic behind this was the observation that fat has 9 kilo-calories (kcal) per gram, whereas protein and carbohydrates have only 4. Therefore, if we cut down on the fat in our diets, we would be consuming fewer calories and thus lose weight. **Well, they were wrong, and what we have today are the results from the longest running prospective cohort study on the effects of diet and obesity, with the public being the cohort.** Imagine that, we were given dietary recommendations without *any* evidence to back them up, and then we became a sort of running experiment which has shown how wrong those recommendations were.

We eat less fat today than 30 years ago, yet we are much, much fatter. What happened? Well, like I mentioned above, when you take something out of the diet, something else has to fill the void. In our case, it was processed carbohydrates of every shape, sort, and flavor. Lots of different low-fat and fat-free junk foods came out to the market, and we were glad to dig in, as long as we didn't touch that steak. I described what happens when foods with a high glycemic load enter the blood – a high level of insulin is secreted, with all of the ensuing harmful effects such as promotion of fat synthesis, prevention of fat burning, etc. Something else happens as well. The large amount of insulin causes too much of the glucose to be taken away from the blood, and the result is a dip in the blood glucose level. The human body likes to keep its glucose levels tightly regulated, and when it senses that dip, you feel tired and HUNGRY. So you eat again. And once again, since fat is pretty much the nutritional equivalent of Satan, you reach for those fat free muffins. In the end, you consume many more calories than you ever would have if you included some fat in your diet. Fat has a satiating effect on the body. It slows down digestion, so that the glucose enters the bloodstream more slowly, with a gentler rise in the amount of insulin secreted and thus a more steady glucose level.

Americans, especially the pediatric and adolescent population, also consume many more sweeteners than in the past. Soda and other sugary beverage consumption has increased dramatically from 30 years ago. To make things worse, the main sweetener used today is high fructose corn syrup. Fructose, despite its low glycemic index, turns out to be a very harmful sugar, increasing triglyceride levels amongst other things. Although fructose is the primary sugar found in fruit, most fruit have a very low amount of sugar and plenty of fiber so that any harmful effect of the fructose is negated.

The bottom line is that to lose weight, following a low-fat diet is not the way to go. Try a hunter-gatherer type diet, such as the TBK Diet, combined with an exercise plan such as the TBK Exercise Program. In hunter-gatherer societies, obesity is unheard of. As people age, they do not become fatter and softer as they do in Western countries, but stay lean.

<u>Osteoporosis</u>

Osteoporosis is extremely common in Western societies amongst the older population, especially women. It is estimated that the lifetime risk for fracture is 40% in women, and 13% in men. In the elderly, a hip fracture can carry a very high risk of death from complications, so osteoporosis is a serious health problem. Unfortunately, most of the guidelines people follow to prevent osteoporosis are rather useless. You have probably heard that in order to prevent osteoporosis, you should obtain plenty of calcium every day (as much as 1200mg for women, and 800mg for men), by eating plenty of dairy foods and/or taking supplements. You might have also been told to perform some weight bearing exercise, especially walking. Some of you might have also heard that vitamin D is important, and others might have been told not to eat too much animal protein. Does all this sound familiar?

Well, it might surprise you that the above advice is not really the way to prevent osteoporosis. For years we have been spoon-fed the idea that the calcium in milk, yogurt, and cheese is essential for building strong bones. Interestingly enough, most of the world is lactose intolerant and can't drink milk, yet still has lower rates of osteoporosis than Western populations in which milk consumption is high. Calcium is only one of the components of bone, but unfortunately, has been pretty much the only one mentioned (largely due to the strong lobbying efforts of the dairy industry). In fact, consuming too much calcium may actually be detrimental to your bones in addition to your health (see my discussion of prostate cancer above).

Furthermore, dairy products, although high in calcium, might not be the best method for protecting your bones. In fact, a large review article from the *American Journal of Clinical Nutrition* concluded that the only subset of people who ***might*** benefit from dairy products in the prevention of osteoporosis is women under 30 years of age. The

41

problem with dairy products is twofold. First, dairy products such as milk and cheese contain high amounts of calcium but low amounts of magnesium, which is also a crucial nutrient in strengthening the skeleton. Thus you get a very high ratio of calcium to magnesium, which can lead to increased urinary loss of magnesium. Second, most calcium containing dairy products, including milk, but especially cheese, also contain significant amounts of sodium. Sodium causes urinary calcium loss, and so you're literally peeing your calcium away, especially if you consume significant amounts of other processed foods like snack foods, processed meats, soy products, and other processed junk foods.

More and more research now supports the idea that protecting your bones is more a function of the amount of calcium that you retain in your bones rather than the amount you consume. Thus eating large amounts of calcium alone won't do the trick. If anything, it will make you deficient in magnesium, which will hurt you in the end. You *should* try to consume adequate amounts of calcium, but dairy might not be optimum. Try increasing your intake of sardines, halibut, ocean perch, pike, trout, canned salmon, almonds, brazil nuts, oranges, prickly pears, blackberries, black currants, figs, kumquats, spinach, leafy greens, and if you want, a cup or so of calcium fortified orange or grapefruit juice. These are all healthy, natural, foods that will ensure good calcium intake without the unhealthy effects of dairy products. Furthermore, they are all good sources of other essential nutrients.

One of those is magnesium, a mineral found in nuts, seeds, vegetables, and in smaller amounts in fruit and meat. Magnesium is essential not only for bone health, as it is one of the components of bone, but also for heart health and the prevention of hypertension. Unfortunately, the vast majority of us who live on processed food are grossly deficient in this essential nutrient, which is contributing to poor health. Potassium, found in high amounts in fruits, vegetables, meat and fish, also is crucial for the prevention of osteoporosis, but not because it is a component of bone, but rather because it is important in preventing urinary losses of calcium and magnesium. As was stated above, preventing urinary losses of calcium, especially as we age, is the key to preventing osteoporosis, and thus eating a diet rich in potassium and low in sodium is of the utmost importance. Indeed, more and more studies are coming out showing that increased intake of fruits and vegetables is protective against osteoporosis.

The next component in our bone health discussion is protein, or more specifically animal protein. Many nutritionists have bashed animal protein, claiming that a high protein diet will cause weak bones because protein can lead to increased urinary excretion of calcium. However, the scientific evidence speaks for itself. **One large study published in the *Journal of Bone and Mineral Research* showed that both elderly men and women who consumed the most *animal* protein had the lowest rate of bone loss, whereas those who consumed little protein had much higher rates of bone loss. Another study published in the *American Journal of Clinical Nutrition* has shown that postmenopausal women (the group of people at highest risk for osteoporosis) who consumed the highest amount of protein, particularly animal protein, had the strongest bones, and were the least likely to suffer from hip fractures.** Other studies have shown similar findings (however, higher intake of vegetable protein does not yield the same benefits as animal protein, and in at least one study is associated with higher risk of fracture). Furthermore, research has shown that low protein diets hamper recovery from fractures (and illness in general).

If we think about it, it makes sense. Bone is a living, active tissue, just like any other in the body. It contains large amounts of cells that are made up partially of protein. A lot of these cells have functions essential to maintaining bone health. Furthermore, eating low amounts of protein usually puts the body in a catabolic state, where muscle is cannibalized for its protein. It could be that in such a state, the body is producing lower amounts of anabolic, bone-building hormones such as testosterone, estrogen, and growth hormone. Our body isn't stupid. Feed it a low amount of protein, and it will channel any that it gets towards essential functions such as keeping essential organs alive at the expense of your muscles, bones, and immune system. And although, as nutritionists point out, protein can cause urinary calcium excretion, it also increases absorption of calcium in the intestine, and the problem of urinary losses can be offset by eating lots of potassium rich fruits and vegetables. Meat and fish contain nice amounts of potassium as well.

The next topic in this discussion is vitamin D, which is essential to calcium absorption in the intestine. In fact, without vitamin D all of the calcium in the world wouldn't be worth anything. Vitamin D may also have a role in the prevention of some cancers. The cheapest, easiest way to get vitamin D is sunlight, which produces vitamin D in your skin. Those of you who shy away from all sunlight, or who always use sunscreen, are doing your body more harm than good. Am I saying you should go out there for hours on end? NO! Of course not. You don't want skin cancer. However, 10-15 minutes a day or more (depending on your skin type) is very healthy. Just don't overdo it or go out around midday when the sun is at its hottest and you'll be fine. Vitamin D is also found in milk, to which it is added, and fatty fish and organ meats. However, all those of you drinking lots of skim milk with your nonfat cereals aren't getting one iota of the vitamin D in the milk since it is a fat soluble vitamin which needs fat to be properly absorbed in the intestine.

The final factor I want to talk about and emphasize, as it is probably one of the most important ones, is weight-bearing exercise. Your body, being efficient, works on a "use it or lose it" mentality. If you sit around all day for 50 years, your body will realize, "Hey, I don't need strong bones or muscles since I never use them! Why waste all this energy trying to maintain them. Let them go to waste and I can go nap." The result is weak muscles and bones, factors that make you more susceptible to fractures. Many people believe that walking is enough to protect you, but I disagree. Walking is a healthy exercise, but I don't believe that the stress on your skeleton is enough to keep those bones strong. Instead, lifting weights or performing calisthenics such as deep knee bends should do the trick.

In conclusion, we have seen that to protect our bodies from getting osteoporosis, we should consume a low sodium diet rich in calcium, magnesium, potassium, animal protein, as well as get some sunlight for vitamin D and perform weight-bearing exercises like weight-lifting or calisthenics. By following a hunter-gatherer type diet such as the TBK diet, rich in fresh fruits and vegetables, fish and fresh meat, you will get all of the above nutrients in natural healthy proportions. Furthermore, by following the TBK Exercise Program, you will build up those bones and muscles.

Autoimmune Disease

There haven't been any studies performed on a hunter-gatherer diet's therapeutic effects on autoimmune diseases such as lupus, rheumatoid arthritis, multiple sclerosis, ulcerative colitis, Crohn's disease and Sjogren's syndrome, but there is some anecdotal evidence suggesting that the avoidance of processed oils (which are high in n-6 fats), grains, dairy products, sugars, legumes, and potatoes might help alleviate some of the symptoms, as well as possibly prevent the disease to begin with. Autoimmune diseases are caused when the body's immune system turns against itself. What happens is part of a virus or bacteria resembles a structure in the body, and so the immune cells end up attacking that particular substance thinking it's the enemy. A similar scenario can happen with certain proteins from food. Although theoretically, proteins are fully digested into amino acids in the stomach and small intestine, in reality, some whole proteins or protein fragments manage to enter the bloodstream from the digestive tract, coming into contact with immune cells. Since some proteins such as casein from milk resemble certain structures in the body, it is possible that the body will end up attacking itself.

<u>Vegetarian Diets</u>

Many people today think that vegetarian diets are the healthiest diets, and that they can prevent heart disease and cancer, in addition to helping save the planet. There are two basic reasons that people follow vegetarian diets – to improve their health and/or because of ethical issues. There is a whole spectrum of different vegetarian diets. On the one end is the vegan diet, in which no animal products are consumed whatsoever. Then there are lacto-ovo vegetarians who eat dairy and eggs (sometimes one but not the other), and then there are people who hardly ever eat meat, those that eat only fish but not poultry or meat, and those that just abstain from red meat.

Let's start off by examining the health benefits of such diets. A study which pooled five large prospective studies found that vegetarians had a 24% lower mortality rate from heart disease than non-vegetarians. However, there was NO statistically significant difference in death rates from stomach cancer, colon cancer, breast cancer, prostate cancer, stroke, and all other causes between vegetarians and non-vegetarians. Furthermore, when you examine the mortality rates from heart disease more closely, you find that in comparison to regular meat eaters, people who occasionally eat meat had a 20% lower mortality rate, people who eat fish but not meat had a 34% lower mortality rate, lacto-ovo vegetarians had a 34% lower mortality rate, and vegans had a 26% lower mortality rate.

Thus, it seems that the exclusion of animal products or saturated fat from the diet was not what protected the vegetarians against heart disease, since the lacto-ovo group, as well as those that ate fish, had much lower rates of heart disease than the vegan group, and even the occasional meat eaters had similar rates to the vegans. In all likelihood, it is the higher consumption of fresh fruits, vegetables, and nuts rather than the exclusion of meat that provides protection against heart disease. As I will discuss below, nuts protect against heart disease, and it is known that vegetarians, who use nuts as a source of protein, consume larger amounts than non-vegetarians. Vegetarians also eat more fruits and vegetables, which also provides protection against heart disease. One can reap the benefits of a vegetarian diet by eating more nuts, fruits, and vegetables instead of excluding animal products from the diet.

There are potentially harmful effects to vegetarian diets, particularly the vegan diets. Since animal products, especially red meat, supply many vitamins and minerals that are tougher to obtain from plant foods, deficiencies can arise. For example, vitamin B-12 is found ONLY in animal products, so vegans are at risk for this type of deficiency, which could result in anemia and nerve damage. Zinc also is found in much higher amounts in meat. Iron from animal products is in a form that is much more readily absorbed in the body than the iron found in plants. The potential iron deficiency that can result from follow a vegan diet is a particular problem in menstruating women, pregnant women, and children. Furthermore, soy, which forms a large part of many vegetarian diets, is quite high in phytic acid, which prevents absorption of many minerals, further exacerbating nutritional deficiencies. Soy also contains a number of enzyme inhibitors that prevent proper digestion of dietary protein, which could also be problematic in children who need high quality protein to grow and properly develop. In addition, following a vegan diet or any other vegetarian diet low in animal protein can ***increase*** your risk for osteoporosis (refer to my discussion of osteoporosis above).

Next, I want to challenge the claim that vegetarians make that their diet is natural. First of all, by virtue of the fact that one cannot obtain vitamin B-12 from a vegan diet means that no hunter-gatherer or other primitive society could have ever followed such a diet since in the absence of vitamin supplements or vitamin fortified foods it would lead to death. Thus, this cannot be the natural diet of human beings. Second, much of the vegetarian cuisine is extremely processed food. For example, tofu is a processed soy product, and all of those soy frozen dinners you find in the supermarket are processed as well, with many containing high levels of sodium and unnatural additives.

Finally, I want to touch upon the ethical dimension of vegetarian diets. The common argument is that eating a vegetarian diet saves animals, as well as the environment, since the cattle used to feed us consume many times more grain than humans do. By not eating cows, we help protect the environment. However, the problem isn't with eating cows. The problem lies with the fact that most cows are fattened with large amounts of grains and soybeans instead of following a natural diet of grasses. If all cattle ranchers raised their cows on grass by letting them graze in the pastures, there would be no need for all of the grains to feed them, and in addition, the meat would be healthier and richer in n-3 fatty acids. Nomads in many parts of the world simply migrate with their herds of goats or sheep from one pasture to the next, allowing the grass to re-grow in between.

If this was the scenario, vegetarian diets would be causing more environmental damage because humans would be the only ones eating grains and soybeans, both ecologically disastrous crops. If humans ate pasture-fed meat, fish, fruits and vegetables and fewer grains, the environment would indeed be better off. It is not fair then to attack eating meat; rather the methods by which the cows are raised. You might wonder, what about the poor cows? Even if they were pasture fed, they would still be killed and eaten. Well, the fact is that producing enough grain to feed human beings who eat no meat would result in the deaths of many more animals, as well as the reduced diversity of animals as a result of turning wilderness areas into cornfields or rice paddies.

Tamir B. Katz, M.D.

Foods You Should Eat on the TBK Diet

Fruit & Berries – apples, oranges, peaches, pears, plums, cherries, grapefruit, cantaloupes, honeydew melons, watermelons, lemons, limes, cherries, apricots, strawberries, blueberries, raspberries, grapes, nectarines, apricots, tangerines, pineapples, papayas, guavas, mangos, bananas, kiwifruit, kumquats, pomegranates, prickly pears, star fruit, currants, dates, figs, olives, avocadoes, tomatoes, and any other raw, edible fruit.

Vegetables – lettuces, cabbages, spinach, any other leafy vegetables, cucumbers, onions, celery, carrots, broccoli, cauliflower, zucchini, radishes, turnips, peppers, scallions, alfalfa sprouts, squash, edible mushrooms, garlic, edible flowers, herbs, and spices, and any other vegetable that can be eaten raw.

Fresh Meat, Poultry, Fish, & Eggs – fresh meat, poultry, fish, organ meats, and eggs. Do NOT eat anything raw from this category because of potential bacterial contamination. Emphasize game meat such as bison or venison, and try to buy leaner cuts of beef. **Avoid shark, swordfish, tilefish, king mackerel, lake trout, bass, marlin, and snapper, as they contain high levels of mercury which can be harmful, especially to young children, infants, and fetuses. Pregnant or nursing women, young children, and toddlers should eat other fish in moderation. Emphasize salmon, cod, haddock, pollock, flounder, Atlantic mackerel, smelt, whitefish, and sardines, which have low mercury levels.** Buy Omega-3 enriched eggs.

Nuts & Seeds – almonds, pecans, filberts (hazelnuts), walnuts, brazil nuts, macadamia nuts, pistachios, hickory nuts, coconuts, pumpkin seeds, sunflower seeds, flax seeds, sesame seeds, tahini, and any other nut or seed that can be eaten raw. Peanuts and cashews are legumes and thus should be avoided. Make sure to buy only raw nuts and seeds, not ones which are cooked in vegetable or seed oils and salted, as is often the case.

Oils – Olive oil – preferably extra virgin grade olive oil as it is the least refined. Coconut oil is also acceptable.

Drinks – drink mostly water. Tea, seltzer, and *small amounts* of fresh squeezed fruit juices or wine are fine as well. Avoid fruit drinks or juices from concentrate. Also don't overdo the herb teas. Most are perfectly harmless, but some such as comfrey can cause liver damage when drunk too often.

Sweeteners – small amounts of honey or maple syrup (but not the commercially available maple syrup which is nothing but corn syrup and coloring – I'm talking about the genuine maple syrup from maple trees).

Other – salsa or other tomato sauces (as long as they contain only allowed ingredients), small amounts of salt (preferably sea salt), small amounts of wine vinegar.

Although you can eat from any of the foods above, don't eat too many dates, figs, raisins, bananas, papayas, fruit juices, or sweeteners, as they are all high in sugar.

There is NO need to count grams of fat, carbohydrates, or calories. Just eat whenever you are hungry. Eat until you are satiated, but not to the point of feeling sick. This is unhealthy as it stretches your stomach and strains your digestive system. **Again, you should never feel hungry on this diet. Anytime you feel hungry, EAT! Just stick with the above foods.**

Before moving on to the foods you should avoid, let's briefly examine the health benefits of the aforementioned foods that you should emphasize. Fresh fruits, berries, and vegetables are high in vitamins, minerals, antioxidants, and fiber, and for the most part have a low glycemic load. They may protect against heart disease, certain cancers, diabetes, and osteoporosis, and thus are an essential part of any healthy diet. Fresh red meat is high in all of the B vitamins, vitamin A, vitamin D, potassium, zinc, highly absorbable iron, magnesium, and is a wonderful source of high quality protein. As we discussed above, processed meat (see below) should be avoided, but fresh meat is a healthy source of many nutrients. Fish also contain many of the same beneficial nutrients as meat, in addition to heart-protective n-3 fatty acids. **Just remember to eat a variety of fish, as eating only large fish can result in potentially harmful mercury levels.** Nuts are the best dietary source of magnesium, which protects the heart through a variety of different mechanisms including prevention of fatal arrhythmias and prevention of arterial calcification, which leads to blocked and weakened arteries. Nuts also contain healthy fats and fiber. Several studies have shown a link between nut consumption and longevity as well as decreased rates of heart disease.

Foods to Avoid

Oils – corn, cottonseed, soybean, safflower, sunflower, vegetable, peanut, canola (rapeseed) oils, cod liver oil, flaxseed oil, margarine, shortening, any product which contains hydrogenated or partially hydrogenated oils (most baked goods and packaged goods), mayonnaise, most packaged salad dressings, and any product which contains any of these oils.

Sweeteners – sugar, corn syrup, high fructose corn syrup, fructose, dextrose, maltose, molasses, sorbitol, saccharin, aspartame, and any products which contain them such as candy, baked goods, frosting, ice cream, and many sauces.

Processed Meats/Fish – hot dogs, sausage, bacon, deli meats/ cold cuts (e.g. pastrami, salami, bologna, ham, corned beef, chicken/ turkey cold cuts), any other cured meat, cured herring, lox, or any other cured fish.

Dairy Products – milk, chocolate milk, cream, all cheeses, butter, ice cream, yogurt, frozen yogurt, sour cream, half and half, pudding, and any other product made with or from dairy.

Grains – flour, cakes, cookies, muffins, scones, donuts, biscuits, crackers, pretzels, pasta, bagels, breads, noodles, macaroni, any other baked goods, breakfast cereals, rice cakes, rice, corn, grits, corn starch, barley, buckwheat, oats, millet, spelt, rye, bran, couscous, wheat germ, anything with batter (most fried foods), corn chips, tortillas, and any other flour or grain product.

Tubers – potatoes, yams, sweet potatoes, cassava, taro, tapioca, potato chips, French fries, potato starch, and any product containing the above.

Legumes – soy, kidney, wax, pinto, lima, navy, black, green, peas, lentils, chick peas, peanuts, cashews, tofu, miso, soy sauce, hummus, coffee, chocolate, and any other bean, legume, or bean product.

Drinks – Sodas (regular or diet), fruit drinks, lemonade, punch, coffee, diet drinks, hard alcohol (e.g. vodka, whisky, rum, gin), beer, fruit juice from concentrate, sweetened ice tea, any other drink made with sugar or corn syrup.

Other – catsup, mustard, duck sauce, vinegar, salt in all but small amounts, packaged foods, canned soups, any product which contains ingredients from the foods to avoid.

Let's briefly look at why the above foods should be avoided. Because the oils mentioned above are high in n-6 and/or *trans* fats they may contribute to the development of heart disease and the progression and growth of tumors, as well as lead to a pro-inflammatory environment in the body. The foods in the sweeteners category, especially high fructose corn syrup, are largely responsible for our current obesity and diabetes epidemics, as well as the development of heart disease and certain cancers, due to the large glycemic load of the foods in which they are found. Processed meats are high in salt and carcinogenic preservatives. Dairy products may increase the risk for prostate cancer. Milk protein and lactose have been very strongly correlated with heart disease, although the mechanism is still unclear. In addition, milk is also a potential cause of type 1 diabetes, certain mental disorders, and testicular cancer.

Refined grains and starches carry a high glycemic load, increasing your risk of developing heart disease, diabetes, certain cancers, and obesity. Furthermore, many foods that contain processed grains also contain *trans* fats, sugar, sodium, and harmful preservatives, stabilizers, and flavor enhancers such as MSG and carrageenan. Most tubers also contain a high glycemic load. In addition, most contain various toxins such as inhibitors of digestive enzymes, and glycoalkaloids, which disrupt cell membranes and cause cancerous changes. It is unknown what proportion of these toxins are deactivated through cooking.

Furthermore, as I discussed above, fried potatoes, chips, breads, and many other cooked starches contain very high levels of the carcinogen acrylamide. Thus, even unrefined breads and certain other grains, although healthier in some respects, are still not so healthy. Legumes, although they carry a medium to low glycemic load, also contain several toxins and enzyme inhibitors. Soy also contains anti-thyroid substances which may decrease one's metabolism, making a person fatter. Indeed, soybeans, along with grains, are used to fatten cattle and pigs in this country. The drinks category contains mostly drinks with a high sugar content, or hard alcohol, which in large amounts can lead to pancreatitis, liver damage, and accidents, including car accidents when people are stupid enough to get behind the wheel while intoxicated.

Vitamins and Supplements

Vitamins and other nutritional supplements are extremely popular today. Millions of Americans use them daily in the hopes of improving their health, and so the topic merits a discussion. I will start off by discussing the antioxidant vitamins – beta-carotene, vitamin C, and vitamin E. People take these mainly in the hopes of preventing heart disease and cancer. There is little to no evidence that antioxidants provide any benefit in preventing either one. In fact, some studies have shown possible adverse effects when megadoses are taken. Furthermore, in smokers, it has been observed that people who take beta-carotene supplements might actually increase their risk of developing lung cancer, although the mechanism is unclear. There *might* be some benefit of antioxidant vitamins in the prevention of Alzheimer's disease. **The bottom line is that eating a diet rich in fresh fruits and vegetables provides all of the antioxidants one needs in *appropriate* doses.**

In nature, vitamins found in plants and animals exist in a certain proportion to other vitamins and substances in the food. Supplements extract one specific form of a vitamin and supply it in unnaturally high doses. Whereas from food, the body absorbs all of the nutrients, the abnormally high concentration of the specific vitamin found in a particular supplement might cause an imbalance, causing the uptake of one vitamin or form of the vitamin at the expense of others. Vitamin E is a good example. It is often sold as alpha-tocopherol, which is only one form of the vitamin. In natural foods, there are many different tocopherols, all of which are important. What happens is that the supplement delivers a huge amount of alpha-tocopherol, which saturates the receptors in the small intestine and causes the absorption of only the one form of the vitamin at the expense of others.

Furthermore, fruits and vegetables contain other beneficial substances besides the actual vitamins. That is why studies have shown that consumption fresh fruits and vegetables may protect against heart disease and certain cancers while obtaining vitamins and antioxidants through supplements does not. In conclusion, based on the current evidence, **I do not recommend taking supplements of the antioxidant vitamins, especially at high doses which might actually be harmful.**

Next I'll discuss B vitamins, which are often sold as a B-complex supplement that provides all of the B-vitamins, in addition to folate. There is solid evidence that these vitamins have cardiovascular benefits, mainly through lowering homocysteine levels as discussed above. Niacin is also used to lower triglycerides. **However, meat, poultry, and fish all contain very nice amounts, so those of you on the TBK Diet do not have to supplement your diet.** However, people who eat very little of these foods, such as vegetarians, or those of you who currently have heart disease, might benefit from a B-complex supplement, **provided you don't take large doses. If the supplement contains more of the vitamin than is recommended by the recommended daily allowance (RDA), do NOT use that supplement** (the amount of the vitamin with respect to the RDA will be listed on the back of the vitamin container – the values shouldn't exceed 100%).

Multivitamins are extremely popular. They contain vitamin A or beta-carotene, vitamin C, vitamin E, vitamin D, all of the B vitamins, and several minerals. Again, those of you on the TBK Diet, or who otherwise eat plenty of fresh fruits, vegetables and fresh meat, poultry, and fish, do not need to take one, but for those of you with a less than adequate diet, it is not a bad idea. There are a few things to watch out for. First of all, do NOT take a multivitamin that supplies megadoses of the vitamins. **Again, look at the back of the container, which will show you how much of the vitamin is present with respect to the RDA. If you see over 100% for several of the vitamins, especially vitamin A and vitamin D, avoid that brand. Also, buy brands that contain no iron, or at the very least have a low amount.** Many foods, including meat and most grains (which in this country are fortified) have a decent amount of iron in them, so it is not a good idea to supplement your diet with more.

Excess iron can be harmful, possibly contributing to heart disease and some cancers. **However, if you are told to take iron by your physician, by all means follow his or her directions.**

Calcium supplements are also extremely popular, especially among women who think it will prevent osteoporosis. As I discussed above, this belief is erroneous. Unless your diet is really awful, there is no need to take calcium supplements. If you still feel obliged, take no more than 300-600mg a day in the form of a supplement (½ the dose with breakfast, ½ with dinner). More than this amount might lead to health problems. Refer back to my discussion of prostate cancer for an explanation.

The one supplement I think most people would benefit from, especially older people or those with heart disease, is magnesium. Although this important, heart protective mineral is found in generous quantities in nuts, and in smaller amounts in meat, fruits, vegetables, and whole grains, those who eat very few nuts or who generally eat a processed food based diet, would benefit from taking up to 500mg a day (250 mg with meals twice a day).

Next on the list of supplements are the plethora of fat burners out there today which contain various substances such as ephedrine that speed up your metabolism. Although many of them work, the potential serious side effects, which include heart problems, psychosis and possibly death, are not worth the benefits. The problem with the newer supplements is that most haven't been around long enough for people to test for any adverse side effects. Thus, as with the diet drug fen-phen which was discovered to damage the heart, the potential side effects of all of these weight loss and diet supplements should not be taken lightly. There are no short cuts or quick fixes in life. If you want to be healthy and in great shape, exercise and follow a proper diet.

Herbal supplement use for various conditions has become very popular in this country. A detailed discussion of all of the herbs out there is beyond the scope of this work, but I will issue the following warnings. Some herbs can interact with a variety of different medications as well as with anesthetics, so always consult your physician before taking them if you are currently on any medications or if you are scheduled for an operation. In particular, HIV positive people should beware because some herbs have the potential to interact with their HIV medications, rendering them less effective. Same thing with patients undergoing chemotherapy for cancer. Don't be stupid and risk your life and health. Another problem with herbs is that in many cases you don't know what you're getting. The FDA is under no legal obligation to regulate supplements and so often times some batches will have a lot of the active ingredients while others will have almost none.

Furthermore, many herbs can have harmful effects on the liver. The fact that traditional healers in China have been using an herb for thousands of years does not make the pill you are about to swallow good for you. The authentic, old time healers knew how much of which part of the plant to use for each individual and for how long (and even then some people were harmed). You should not take it upon yourselves to decide which herbs treat what. Although studies have shown that some herbs/plants have beneficial properties (e.g. saw palmetto berry for benign prostate hypertrophy, St. John's wort for depression), in MOST cases herbs have not undergone rigorous studies to determine their long term safety or efficacy. **The bottom line is that I think you should AVOID herbal supplements. The potential benefits are few, while the potential side effects, especially for those with pre-existing illnesses, are numerous.**

Finally, I would like to touch upon the use of aspirin in disease prevention. Aspirin has been shown to work wonders for those at high risk of suffering a heart attack or stroke, and recent studies have shown that it may protect against colon cancer as well. **However, aspirin can have serious side effects in certain people, especially in children to whom it should never be given without permission of a physician. Before deciding to take an aspirin, consult with your physician if it's for you. For the average, healthy man or woman, the possible side effects probably outweigh the benefits.**

Food Shopping

The key to successful eating starts at your local supermarket. In this section, I will show you how to go about purchasing the food which is the cornerstone of the TBK diet.

Start off in the produce section. Stock up on any of the aforementioned fruits, vegetables, nuts and seeds. Avoid canned fruits and vegetables, opting for fresh, raw produce. If you can afford it, buy organic produce, which is free of pesticides. Either way, wash your produce well before consumption.

Buy only **RAW** nuts and seeds. Almost all of the roasted ones are cooked in harmful vegetable oils and have a high salt content. Read the ingredients, choosing only products that have the nut or seed as the only ingredient. Preferably buy whole nuts in the shell. Freeze any nuts and seeds that you're not going to eat within the next few days to keep them fresh and inhibit mold growth.

If you have a sweet tooth, stock up on some dried fruit such as raisins, apricots, figs, and dates. Again, read the labels. The only ingredient should be the dried fruit. Unfortunately, **most dried fruit is preserved with sulfites or other preservatives,** so again, be vigilant and read the labels.

Finally, to ensure lower costs and fresher produce, purchase fruits and vegetables that are in season.

Next, move on to the meat aisle. Emphasize leaner cuts of meat, and make sure the meat and poultry look fresh. If your supermarket offers it, game meat such as bison or venison is healthier. **Avoid deli meats, cured meats, hot dogs, sausages, and bacon. Most contain nitrites and other harmful preservatives and/or binding agents, and even those that don't have a large amount of salt.** Frozen meat and poultry are fine as well, but avoid freezer burned products, indicated by excessive ice formation or discoloration.

On to the fish section. Purchase nice looking fish that do not have a strong fishy smell, an indication of spoilage. Frozen fish is also fine, but avoid freezer burned ones, often indicated by excessive ice formation on the fish. Try to buy ocean fish as opposed to farm raised fish, since the latter are often fed grains, which decreases their n-3 fatty acid levels and increases their n-6 fatty acid levels. Often times, the fish won't be labeled, so ask the people who work at the store.

Canned fish are fine as well, especially sardines and mackerel, but again, you must read the labels. Canned fish such as tuna and sardines are often packaged in unhealthy vegetable oils, and often contain such harmful additives as hydrolyzed soy or vegetable proteins, vegetable broth and/or other preservatives and flavor enhancers. Look for products that contain only fish and water (salt is okay if you can't find unsalted products or do not like the taste). Products packed in olive oil are fine as well. Add spices, lemon juice, and herbs at home to flavor it.

Canned sardines and mackerel packed in water are amongst the healthiest fish to eat as they contain a nice dose of healthy Omega-3 fat as well as high quality protein and some calcium. Furthermore, they are small fish which are lower down on the food chain and therefore have a lower concentration of mercury and other contaminants than larger fish.

Next comes juice. I suggest you squeeze your own fresh juices, but for convenience, not-from-concentrate juices are acceptable once in a while. This means 100% juice with no added water, preservatives, or sugar.

Almost done. All you need now are a few odds and ends. Go to the oil section and pick out some extra virgin olive oil. If you dislike its taste, buy regular olive oil, but try to avoid light olive oil which is more highly processed. Finally, stock up on different spices. Once again, check the ingredients, since some spices contain potentially harmful additives. Purchase only products that have the spice as the only ingredient.

There, you are done. Wasn't so bad was it? Next we'll look at how to start the diet.

How to Start

Now that you know what to eat and what to buy, it's time to take action and begin changing your eating habits. You might not be able to switch cold turkey to the TBK Diet, but that's okay. A gradual change in eating habits might, in the long run, help you stick to the diet. One way to do it is as follows, but any way that works for you is perfectly fine.

Step 1

Start by drastically cutting down or even eliminating the junk food in your diet. Avoid cookies, cakes, crackers, donuts, pretzels, chips, muffins, candy, ice cream, etc. Make sure not to keep junk food at home lest you be tempted to indulge. If you want a snack, try a piece of fresh fruit, some raw nuts, or a small sandwich.

Step 2

A couple of weeks after step 1, begin replacing the processed foods you eat during the meals with less processed or unprocessed ones. For example, instead of eating a refined breakfast cereal, have a bowl of oatmeal made from whole rolled oats (not the instant variety). Instead of white bread, switch to a coarse whole grain bread. Also, begin replacing some of the starchy side dishes you eat, such as potatoes or pasta, with vegetables such as broccoli, asparagus, cauliflower, etc. For dessert, try half a cantaloupe topped with strawberries. Have some fresh fruit instead of a "health" muffin which is loaded with sugar and unhealthy fats.

Step 3

A couple of weeks after implementing step 2, begin step 3. You have probably lost some weight by now, especially if you have been exercising. Eliminate milk from your diet, sticking to cheese and small amounts of butter. Furthermore, after your lunch meal, eat only foods which are on the TBK Diet.

Step 4

A couple of weeks after step 3, initiate step 4 by continuing what you have been doing, in addition to adding 3 days a week in which you are completely on the TBK diet.

Step 5

Switch completely to the TBK diet a couple of weeks after step 4. If you want to, give yourself a day off once a week in which you eat what you want *within limit.* Don't go wolfing down a box of donuts and 2 pizzas. Include some healthy food on your off day as well, and eat normal sized meals.

The key to sticking with the TBK diet is to make your food as appetizing as possible. Try out different recipes. Be creative! Use different spices, seasonings, herbs, etc. The TBK Diet might seem bland at first because your body is used to being inundated with strong flavors of sweet and salty from all of the processed foods and flavor enhancers you've been eating. But stick with it, and you'll realize how luscious a cold juicy orange is or how mouth watering a grilled piece of fish which has been marinating in lemon juice, extra virgin olive oil, and spices is. After all, can that freezer meal you've called dinner really compete with what nature has provided?

Cooking and Food Preparation

Cooking and preparing your own food is the way to go, since you know exactly what is going into your food, and that (hopefully) the food you are going to be ingesting is handled and prepared in a clean and hygienic manner. Below are some tips on cooking and handling your food, as well as how to save time.

When cooking, boil, bake, broil, roast, or grill, but **avoid frying**. Sautéing is okay as well. Avoid charring your food or otherwise overcooking it.

Handle your raw meat, poultry, fish, and eggs with great care so that you don't contaminate counter tops or other kitchen fixtures. Make sure to thoroughly wash any surface, dish, or utensil that has come into contact with raw meat, poultry, fish, or eggs.

Cooking and preparing your own food can take a lot of time if done on a daily basis. My suggestion to you is to pick one or two cooking nights per week, prepare the meals then, and either freeze them or put them in the fridge for later re-heating and consumption. **However, do NOT reheat foods containing meat, poultry, fish, or eggs more than once because of potential bacterial contamination.** Reheat only the portion that you want to eat at the moment, leaving the rest in the fridge or freezer.

The most important thing is to keep it interesting. Cook with a loved one. Try different recipes out. Marinate meat in red wine, extra virgin olive oil, and garlic, and fish such as salmon in extra virgin olive oil, pepper and lemon juice, or use any marinades you enjoy from ingredients on the TBK Diet. Grow your own vegetables and herbs. Keep it fun.

Eating Out

Although it is best to prepare your own meals, there will be times when you must eat out. For some of you, this might be every single day. In this section, I will provide some tips on how to eat out while staying on the TBK Diet. The basic rules are the same. Stick to the allowed foods. Make sure to ask about the ingredients in the different dishes you eat. Many sauces and dressings contain sugars and harmful oils. Many soups and stews use flour or starch as thickeners, and some will have milk in them as well. Also, restaurants often use cheap vegetable oils and/or margarine when cooking instead of olive oil. Watch out for cooked vegetables and fried or scrambled eggs, which are often cooked in vegetable oils. Be vigilant, because you could easily be eating harmful foods which have the same appearance as the healthy foods you cook at home.

You should find things to eat at most types of restaurants. In a diner, you can get steaks, roasts, chicken, fish, salad, hard boiled eggs, and fruit. In most fast food places, you can get a grilled chicken sandwich and a hamburger which you can eat without the bun. Many fast food places today offer salads as well. Many restaurants will let you make substitutions. For example, if your steak comes with fries and a small salad, many places will allow you to have a double portion of salad instead of the fries. Furthermore, many places will offer you a choice in method of preparation, for example they will allow you to order steamed vegetables instead of ones sautéed in vegetable oil. Go for grilled, steamed, baked, or roasted instead of fried. Most restaurants, whether Italian, Mexican, Chinese, Japanese, deli, or American type cuisines, will have some kind of fresh meat, fish, or poultry, and some type of salad or vegetable dish.

Breakfast can be more problematic. Bacon and sausage are not good choices because they are cured, salty, processed meats. Fried eggs are not a great choice either because, as I mentioned above, cheap, unhealthy oils are often used. In addition, frying in and of itself

is not healthy. You might be able to get hard boiled eggs or p
eggs in some places. If not, eat a lighter breakfast of different
and nuts, and have your larger, meat or fish based meals for lunch a
dinner.

Sample Meals

Below, several sample meals and snacks are provided to give you an idea of what to make and eat. This is by no means a comprehensive list or menu nor is it intended to be one – you should create your own meals or modify recipes in magazines or cookbooks using ingredients allowed by the TBK Diet.

Sample Breakfasts:

1. Steak (marinated overnight in extra virgin olive oil, red wine, garlic) and eggs with ½ grapefruit.

2. Omelet with 2-3 eggs, raw peppers, onions, mushrooms, tomatoes, spices, a touch of salt, olive oil, half a cantaloupe topped with strawberries, 1 small glass of fresh squeezed grapefruit juice.

3. Cereal – combine chopped pecans, walnuts, hazelnuts, almonds, apples, dates, bananas, prunes, peaches and/or coconut in a bowl. Add some cinnamon, a couple of tablespoons of honey and a tablespoon of orange juice. Add a small amount of coconut or almond milk and enjoy! For a hot cereal, simply heat the above mixture in a small skillet. Alternatively, you can make your own cereal with any fruit and nut combination that you enjoy. Experiment and have fun!

4. Cold salmon cooked with a dash of salt and pepper, with a squeeze of lemon on top, fruit salad of apples, oranges, pears, peaches, cherries, cup of tea.

Sample Lunches:

1. Large vegetable salad with a tin of sardines, hard boiled egg, lettuce, tomatoes, onions, avocado, cucumbers, topped with an extra virgin olive oil, garlic, and lemon juice dressing, orange slices for dessert.

2. Chef salad with pieces of grilled chicken, roast beef, different lettuces, olive oil, garlic, and lemon juice dressing, piece of fruit in season for dessert.

3. Baked cod or any other fish with broccoli or brussel sprouts, large salad, fruit salad topped with shredded coconut for dessert.

4. Beef or lamb stew – beef or lamb cubes, zucchini, tomatoes, onions, celery, mushrooms, carrots, spices, left over chicken or vegetable soup for flavor (optional), cup of tea.

Sample Dinners:

1. Meatballs made from ground beef, buffalo, lamb, chicken, or turkey, a few tablespoons of nut flour, spices, a little salt, cooked in tomato sauce (if from the store, make sure there is no sugar or other forbidden ingredients), sautéed vegetables (celery, onions, broccoli, carrots), frozen grapes for dessert.

2. Barbequed steak, lamb chops, chicken, or fish (make your own BBQ sauce from tomatoes, orange juice, honey, salt, and spices or buy a brand that doesn't have sugar and preservatives), grilled onions, mushrooms, peppers, tomatoes and/or zucchini, large vegetable salad, fresh squeezed fruit juice ice pops for dessert.

3. Stuffed chicken (use celery, mushrooms, ground nuts, carrots, onions and spices for the stuffing, portabello mushrooms sautéed in olive oil and garlic, vegetable patties (shred

zucchini, carrots, onions, carrots, add salt and pepper, combine with egg and nut flour into a patty, and bake in the oven), fruit platter for dessert.

4. Beef brisket with onions and mushrooms, chicken soup, stuffed cabbage (stuff cabbage leaves with ground beef, sautéed onions, egg, spices, and raisins (optional), cook in tomato sauce in oven), glass of red wine, stewed fruit with cinnamon (no sugar) for dessert.

Sample Snacks:

1. Fresh Fruit

2. Fresh veggie sticks (with salsa if you like)

3. Trail mix (any raw nut and dried fruit combo)

4. Cold roast beef slices with veggies

5. Tin of sardines or mackerel with vegetable slices and salsa

6. Smoothie (blend a banana, peach or nectarine, strawberries, (or any fruit combo you like) with crushed ice in a blender)

The TBK Fat Loss Diet

Adopting the TBK Diet will result in improved health and decrease your chances of developing heart disease, diabetes, certain cancers, and osteoporosis. In this section, I will show you how to fine tune the diet to achieve an amazing amount of fat loss.

However, to maximize results and to keep the fat loss permanent, it is imperative that you adopt the TBK Exercise Program (or another effective exercise program) as well.

In addition to adopting the TBK Diet, if you wish to lose fat, avoid dates, figs, raisins and other dried fruit, bananas, papayas, and all fruit juices. In addition, cut down your nut intake by a half, and use less olive oil. Of course, avoid sweets, harmful oils, grains, dairy, tubers, and legumes, and any other harmful foods mentioned above.

There are other tips you can follow. For example, drink 1-2 glasses of water before each meal. If you usually take an "off" day once a week in which you eat what you want, either skip your off day entirely, or else limit yourself to only one meal of whatever you want instead of an entire day.

That's it! No tricks. No complicated routines. No need to count calories, grams of fat or grams of carbohydrates. Even if you simply adopt the TBK Diet and Exercise program without any of the changes suggested in this section, you will still lose weight. These changes are simply provided to speed things up.

The TBK Weight Gain Diet for Underweight People

If you are underweight (skinny), your main goal is to pack on muscle. Eating tons of junk food will make you gain weight, but not the kind of weight you want to gain. You'll just become fat, doughy, and unhealthy. In order to pack on muscle, exercise is very important. No diet in the world will build muscle without exercise. The TBK Exercise Program will build a lot of muscle, especially when you focus on the more advanced exercises. You can also lift weights, but make sure to focus on compound movements such as deadlifts, squats, cleans, snatches, overhead presses, bench presses, and rows. **Have an experienced lifter show you how to lift with good form.** Avoid exercise machines, which tend to be pretty useless for increasing muscle mass. **Eat plenty of fresh meat, fish, fruit (including dried fruit and fresh squeezed juices), nuts, and seeds.**

The Less Strict Diet

Although ideally all of you would stick to the TBK Diet in its entirety and thus obtain the best health and results, I'm a realistic guy, and realize that many of you won't. Therefore, I wrote this section with you in mind. If you follow the advice here, you will still be eating a healthier diet than most Americans. **However, the further you deviate from the TBK diet, the worse your results will be.** Even if you decide to follow a less strict diet, **still emphasize the foods in the TBK diet such as fresh fruits, vegetables, berries, nuts, fresh meat, poultry, and fish.**

On the less strict diet, you may include several foods from the "Foods to Avoid" section. You may include **small amounts** of any of the unprocessed foods listed in the Legume category, but **stay away from processed food** like tofu, most frozen soy products, and any other food that does not resemble the bean from whence it came. From the Tuber category, you may include the **occasional** yam or sweet potato, but still **stay away from regular potatoes** and any products made from them. From the Dairy category, you can include **small amounts** of cheese, butter, cream, and whole milk yogurt (stay away from the supermarket type of yogurt which is loaded with sugar). **Avoid milk, ice cream, chocolate milk, and other dairy products.** Also, make sure any of the above dairy products you buy do NOT include **carrageenan**, a potentially harmful additive found in many dairy products (especially cream, half and half, and ice creams). From the Grains category, include **small amounts** of only unrefined, whole grains such as fresh ears of corn, rolled oats, and coarse whole grain bread with seeds. Avoid all white flour products, and all of the refined grain products such as baked goods, pretzels, crackers, bagels, pasta, etc. Avoid rice as well. From the drinks category, you can have the **occasional** beer.

Avoid all products from the Oils, Sweetener, and Processed Meat categories. Also, generally avoid boxed, packaged, processed food, and salty food.

Note that I emphasize a small amount. How much is a small amount? Well, the less the better. Other than that, you have to use your own judgment. **Don't overdo the grain category because even unrefined grains are fattening in large amounts.**

Another strategy which I mentioned above was to have one "off" day a week where you eat what you want within limits. That is the strategy I use, and it has worked well for me.

The TBK Diet & Children

The TBK diet, the healthiest way for adults to eat, is also the healthiest way for children and adolescents to eat. However, some points need to be emphasized.

Newborns and babies *should* be preferably breastfed or at the very least provided with formula. Coconut, almond, or other nut milks are NOT acceptable alternatives! Although dairy products are not part of the TBK diet, hunter-gatherer babies *are* breastfed. Mother's milk is VERY important for babies and toddlers. You should only start cutting out dairy products at around the age of 3-4.

The first question a lot of you might have is from where can children obtain calcium if they avoid dairy products? As I mentioned above, there is no evidence that children, or anyone for that matter, need tons of calcium to build up their bones. 500-600 mg tops is plenty. That full amount is obtainable by eating a variety of foods on the TBK diet, since many vegetables, fruit, nuts, seeds, and fish contain calcium. However, since children can be picky eaters, providing them with a cup or so a day of calcium fortified orange or grapefruit juice is a good idea. It has as much calcium as milk, and together with the calcium intake from other foods, should ensure more than adequate intake. Furthermore, most children like orange juice so there shouldn't be a problem.

A bigger problem is how to keep the children on the diet while their friends, peers, and even other family members are eating junk food. One way is to get the child used to a healthy diet at an early age. People from various countries often enjoy the food from their country of origin because they were raised on it and are therefore used to that particular cuisine.

Another, more important method to keep your child on a healthy diet is to make the food tasty and appealing. I cannot overemphasize this point. Just think, you are competing with sugar, salt, and flavor enhancer filled snacks, pizza, fries, peanut butter and jelly sandwiches, cookies, candy, etc. Making the food as appetizing as possible is of the utmost importance.

Unfortunately, despite all of your efforts, your child might still crave junk food. If that is the case, allow him or her one day a week when they are off of the diet and provide them with some junk. When you buy junk, or any other food off of the diet, make sure it has no preservatives, **hydrogenated oils**, **carrageenan**, and other chemicals. Generally, the more ingredients found in a food product, the worse it is for you. Also, if you have a tough time pronouncing an ingredient, it's probably also artificial.

One last suggestion is to have your children follow the Less Strict Diet discussed above. It is not as healthy as the full TBK diet, but your child will still be eating much healthier than most other children.

Part 2 – The TBK Exercise Program

Before beginning any exercise program, it is important that you get a complete physical from your physician, *especially* if you are over the age of 35, have any pre-existing heart condition, diabetes, high blood pressure, blood clotting problems, anemia, hernias, joint problems, back problems, a family history of sudden death at a young age, if you smoke, if you are overweight, if you are pregnant, and/or if you haven't exercised in a while (or ever). If you feel any dizziness, chest pain or discomfort, numbness, excessive fatigue or shortness of breath, pain or other severe discomfort while exercising, stop the exercise immediately and call a physician.

Tamir B. Katz, M.D.

Introduction

Exercise is essential to a successful fitness program, whatever your goals are. Most weight loss that is accomplished through diet alone is transient. Furthermore, exercise has several health benefits, including improved cholesterol levels, improved fasting glucose and insulin levels, improved blood pressure, and stronger, denser bones. In fact, a good diet goes a long way towards keeping your bones healthy, but without exercise, specifically weight-bearing exercise such as calisthenics, osteoporosis is still likely.

All of the exercises presented in this section are bodyweight exercises which require no equipment of any kind. There are several advantages to this type of workout. It is very convenient. It can be done anywhere, anytime. Whether you are a businessman who is always on the road, the renter of a tiny apartment with no room for exercise equipment, a college student living in a dormitory, or someone living in a polluted city with no parks or other outdoor recreation areas, you have no excuse not to exercise.

The second advantage is cost. Your own body costs you NOTHING to use. Gym memberships, on the other hand, can be pretty expensive. Most exercise equipment is also very costly. Treadmills cost a fortune, as do weight machines, ab machines, step machines, and even free weights. Furthermore, with most fitness equipment (free weights being the exception), you can only do one type of exercise or workout. The only thing you can do with an ab machine is a crunch type exercise. The only thing you can do with an exercise bicycle is sit and bike. Thus, the real cost of working out with equipment is even higher, since you would have to buy several pieces to obtain a comprehensive workout. But with your own body, you can literally do dozens of different exercises to target all of the muscles of the body, in addition to improving cardiovascular fitness and flexibility.

Another advantage is time efficiency. A bodyweight type workout performed in a circuit fashion (one exercise after the other) can improve strength, muscular endurance, flexibility, and cardiovascular fitness simultaneously. No piece of equipment can do that. A treadmill, step machine, or exercise bike will mainly improve cardiovascular fitness, whereas a weight machine or free weights will mainly improve strength. Therefore your workouts would have to be longer, not to mention the fact that they would not be accomplishing much in the way of improving muscular endurance or flexibility. It is true that you can set up a circuit with the machines at the gym, but the fact that machines tend to isolate muscles instead of working them in unison, coupled with the fact that they are balanced and thus eliminate accessory muscle use, makes them inferior to both free weights and bodyweight exercises in terms of producing functional strength, speed, or muscular endurance. Working out on a leg extension machine only makes you proficient at doing leg extensions, whereas doing 100 deep knee bends will enable you to become more explosive, run faster, kick harder, and lift up heavier objects from the ground.

Bodyweight exercises help develop muscular endurance more than any other type of workout. Muscular endurance is the ability of a muscle to perform at moderate intensity over long periods of time, and it is probably the most useful attribute in everyday scenarios. Carrying small children or bags of groceries, painting a long fence, moving a large volume of furniture and/or boxes, wrestling, practicing other types of martial arts, hiking up a steep mountain with a weighted backpack, shoveling snow, sawing, chopping wood, and horseback riding are all activities that require high levels of muscular endurance. Someone who can bench press 500 pounds but lacks muscular endurance, or someone who can run 10 miles but lacks in the strength department will not be able to sustain many of the aforementioned activities for any length of time.

Finally, bodyweight type routines are probably the safest kind of workout. It is true that free weights are rather safe as well, but the consequences of an accident while lifting weights are usually more severe than when you lift your own bodyweight. Dropping a weight can not only break your foot, but if you are working out at home, the floor will take a pounding as well. In exercises such as the squat and bench press, a workout partner is almost always a must, since getting pinned under a heavy weight can be a disaster. The worse that will happen with a bodyweight exercise (assuming you don't do something stupid like exercise while drunk), is an overuse injury from doing too many repetitions of an exercise resulting in some joint discomfort. In repetitive exercises such as jogging or stair climbing, an overuse injury is almost guaranteed since you are repeating the same motion, often on the same surface, thousands of times. Bodyweight exercises are also performed many times, but not to the same extent. Once you can perform 100 or more repetitions of most exercises, you should switch to a more difficult exercise, thus ensuring the prevention of injury.

Are there any disadvantages to bodyweight only regimens? It is true that to obtain monstrous size, weights are *usually* better (provided you don't waste your time on worthless movements and exercise machines). However, is it a disadvantage not to be enormous? Probably not. In fact, being too big, even if the extra weight is muscle and not fat, might put an unhealthy strain on the body. Furthermore, bodyweight exercises *will* build a large amount of muscle, especially when you follow a proper diet and focus on the more advanced exercises such as handstand push-ups.

Another possible disadvantage that many people cite is difficulty of progression. The argument is that anyone in decent shape will be able to work up to 50 or more push-ups, and unlike free weight exercises, where you can add more weight, you are stuck with your own bodyweight. However, that argument is completely false. If you can do 50 push-ups, try doing them with your legs elevated, or on your knuckles. How many can you do then? How about handstand push-ups. Find me a person who can do 50 straight handstand push-ups, and I'll bet you that person has a more muscular, stronger upper body than most bodybuilders. The same is true for most of the other exercises. If you can do many toe touches, do twisting toe touches. If you can do many calf raises, do them one leg at a time.

In conclusion, there are many advantages to a bodyweight type exercise routine, including convenience, cost effectiveness, development of strength, muscular endurance, flexibility, and cardiovascular fitness in a relatively short workout (which is a huge advantage in today's busy world) with the safe nature of such exercise. There are no real disadvantages of bodyweight routines to any other type of workout.

I have included *over 60* exercises of different degrees of difficulty and for different muscle groups. There are a few reasons for having so many different exercises. One is to avoid boredom. If you had to perform the same exercises all of the time, the routine might get stale and might lead you to neglect your regimen. Another reason is that each one of us is built differently, and so an exercise that might suit me well will not feel right to you, or might be impossible for you to do at your current fitness level. **However, you should NOT avoid exercises simply because they are difficult or because that particular muscle group is weak. If you only do exercises that work muscles which are already strong and neglect your weaker muscle groups you will end up with an unbalanced physique.**

Below are several routines, followed by all of the exercises listed in alphabetical order for easy reference. For optimal results, follow one or more of the core routines, and add any additional exercises you want to round off your routine. However, even if you decide to do only the core routines with no other exercise whatsoever, you will still achieve great results.

No separate warm-up is required. To warm-up, simply perform the first few repetitions of the first and/or second exercise in your routine at a slower pace until you feel the blood entering your muscles and loosening them up. **Do NOT start a routine with Toe Touches, Twisting Instep Touches, Front Kicks, Side Kicks, or Forward Bends.** Doing those exercises without being warmed up could result in a pulled muscle.

When doing an exercise for the first few times, perform it slowly until you have figured it out and can use good form. Sloppy form can lead to injury. Also, read the directions and look at the pictures carefully before doing the exercise, and if it looks significantly more challenging than what you can currently do, skip it and do an easier exercise. With persistence, you will slowly built up to a fitness level at which you will be able to do all of the exercises.

Whatever routine or exercises you choose, the most important thing is to STICK WITH YOUR PROGRAM. Persistence and consistency are the keys to achieving success.

On many of the exercises, I have included a pace at which to do the exercise. As I stated above, start off slowly until you get the hang of the exercise, and gradually build up to the suggested pace. **Always stay in control and use good form.** On many exercises I didn't include a pace for various reasons. Do those exercises at your own pace. **However, do NOT do any of the exercises in slow motion.**

Core Routines

Below are various suggested routines, which through experimentation on myself and others, have found to yield very good results. Some take only minutes a day, whereas others take longer. You should not go over 30-45 minutes on any of the routines. If you find that you are exercising for longer than this, switch to a more advance routine.

When performing the routines below, do each exercise until that particular muscle group is fatigued, but do NOT continue to the point where you can't do another one and are excessively straining.

The most important thing to remember when doing the routines is NOT to rest between the exercises – rather to go onto the next exercise as soon as you are done with the previous one. For example, if your routine consists of Push-ups, followed by Deep Knee Bends, followed by Push-ups again, as soon as you finish the first set of Push-ups, immediately begin the Deep Knee Bends, and as soon as you finish those, do the last set of Push-ups.

Follow the routines below as written. I have arranged the order of the exercises in a specific way to yield optimal results. However, nothing is set in stone. Feel free to make up your own routines, or even try out different exercises. Remember, your own body is unique, and once you develop awareness of it through exercise, you will discover which routines and exercises work best for you.

Work out 5-6 days a week. You can do the same core routine every day, or if you like, follow up to 2 or 3 different core routines a week. If you are following two routines, do one of them on days 1, 3 and 5, and the second one on days 2, 4 and 6. If you are following three core routines each week, do the first one on days 1 and 4, the second one on days 2 and 5, and the third one on days 3 and 6.

If you are sore, do a lighter version of your workout by doing the exercises fewer times than usual, but do NOT skip the workout. If you don't have much time to work out, follow an abbreviated routine, and do a little more on the weekends. But even if you have to wake up 10 minutes earlier every day to fit in your routine, do it. For most of us, such a shortage of time isn't the case. If we honestly examine our lives, we will find that we all have at *least* 5 – 10 minutes a day, often times much more.

Every week or few days, try to increase the number of times you do each exercise. For example, if last week you were doing 50 Deep Knee Bends, try to increase that number to 51 or 52 this week. 100-150 is a good number to aim for. More than that, you might start developing overuse injuries. Once you can do this many repetitions in an exercise, move on to a more difficult exercise, or if you are happy with your current fitness level, simply continue with what you are doing, switching routines once in a while to keep things fresh.

However, 100-150 is an arbitrary number. Some of you will be able to do more, some less. Listen to your own bodies and decide for yourselves. On exercises such as Alternate Punching, Arm Crossovers, Arm Swings, Rowing, Running in Place, Upper Body Sprints, and Upper Cuts, you can go for a few hundred repetitions because of the lower intensity level of these exercises.

While doing the Cat Stretch, Flat Bridge, Leg Grasp, Stationary Squat, T-stance, or Wrestler's Bridge, you are holding a certain position for a length of time, not doing many repetitions of the exercise. For those exercises, increase the amount of time you are holding it. For example, if last week you were holding a Cat Stretch for 30 seconds, try to increase it to 31 or 32 seconds. 2 minutes or more is a good goal to aim for when doing these exercises.

Core Routine 1 – This is the general routine to follow for optimal results. It targets all of the muscles of the body extremely well.

1. Push-ups OR Modified Push-ups OR Standing Push-ups OR Knuckle Push-ups OR Jackknife Push-ups

2. Deep Knee Bends OR Lunges OR Advanced Deep Knee Bends

3. Push-ups OR Modified Push-ups OR Standing Push-ups OR Knuckle Push-ups OR Jackknife Push-ups

4. Toe Touches OR Twisting Instep Touches

5. Push-ups OR Modified Push-ups OR Standing Push-ups OR Knuckle Push-ups OR Jackknife Push-ups

6. Resistance Neck Exercise OR Neck Swings OR Neck Raises

7. Leg Pulls OR Leg Grasp

8. **Deep Breathing Exercise** – pick any of the four that you like

Core Routine 2 – This is an abbreviated routine for those with very little time on their hands.

1. Push-ups OR Modified Push-ups OR Standing Push-ups OR Knuckle Push-ups OR Jackknife Push-ups

2. Deep Knee Bends OR Floor Touches OR One-arm Floor Touches

3. Push-ups OR Modified Push-ups OR Standing Push-ups OR Knuckle Push-ups OR Jackknife Push-ups

4. Bend over and touch your toes (or as close as you can get to them) without bending your knees. Hold the stretch for 20-30 seconds.

Core Routine 3 – This routine is for those who want to be lean and fit, but with less upper body muscle mass.

1. Arm Swings

2. Deep Knee Bends

3. Resistance Neck Exercise

4. Toe Touches OR Twisting Instep Touches

5. **Deep Breathing Exercise** – pick any of the four that you like

Core Routine 4 – The "Deck of Cards" Routine

The "Deck of Cards" routine is used by Japanese wrestlers to get into shape. It is very effective in increasing strength, muscular endurance, and cardiovascular fitness in a relatively short amount of time. Add some stretching at the end of the routine.

The basic workout, as performed by the Japanese, consists of assigning black cards to push-ups, and red cards to deep knee bends. The deck is shuffled, and one draws a card. If for example, a black seven is drawn, 7 push-ups are performed. Similarly, a red nine would mean 9 deep knee bends. All face cards are assigned a value of 10, aces 1 or 11, and a joker 15, 20, 25, or 30 (take you pick). A well conditioned athlete can complete the deck in about 30 minutes or less.

Different variations can be used with the above workout. For example, instead of two exercises, four can be used – one each for spades, hearts, diamonds, and clubs. An example of such a workout would be deep knee bends, push-ups, squat-thrusts, and toe touches. You can up the intensity a bit by performing twice as many deep knee bends as the card value says. If you cannot get through the entire deck, it's okay. Start out by taking out the face cards, and go through the modified deck. The following week, add the four jacks, and so on and so forth until you're doing the entire deck. Beginners can start with the 2's, 3's, 4's, 5's, and 6's, every week or so adding an additional card until they are doing the entire deck.

Perform this routine 3-4 times a week with a day of lighter exercise or rest in between. Below are a few sample routines you can try, but feel free to make up your own. Be creative and have fun with this.

Routine 1

Black Cards – Push-ups OR Modified Push-ups OR Standing Push-ups OR Knuckle Push-ups OR Jackknife Push-ups

Red Cards – Deep Knee Bends OR Floor Touches OR One-arm Floor Touches

Routine 2

Black Cards – Push-ups OR Modified Push-ups OR Standing Push-ups OR Knuckle Push-ups OR Jackknife Push-ups

Red Cards – Leg Pull-in/Extensions

Routine 3

Spades – Push-ups OR Modified Push-ups OR Standing Push-ups OR Knuckle Push-ups OR Jackknife Push-ups

Hearts –Deep Knee Bends OR Lunges

Diamonds – Swing Thrus OR Toe Touches OR Forward Bends

Clubs – Leg Pull-in/Extensions

Routine 4

Spades – Push-ups OR Modified Push-ups OR Standing Push-ups OR Knuckle Push-ups OR Jackknife Push-ups

Hearts – Deep Knee Bends OR Lunges

Diamonds – Squat Thrusts OR Burpees

Clubs – Toe Touches

Routine 5

Spades – Push-ups OR Modified Push-ups OR Standing Push-ups OR Knuckle Push-ups OR Jackknife Push-ups

Hearts – Front Kicks

Diamonds – Side Kicks

Clubs – Deep Knee Bends OR Floor Touches OR One-arm Floor Touches

Core Routine 5 – This routine should be used by those of you who are very overweight as their first routine. **Do NOT attempt to try any intense calisthenics from the beginning, because you may get injured.** Once you have lost weight with the following exercises combined with the TBK Diet, then you can move on to a more challenging regimen.

1. Resistance Neck Exercise

2. Arm Swings

3. Knee Raises

4. Rowing

5. Pelvic Lifts

6. Arm Crossovers

7. **Deep Breathing Exercise** – pick any of the four that you like

8. **Walking** – 15-30 minutes

Core Routine 6 – This routine is for maximal fat loss and a great set of abs. Do it twice a day, and make sure to follow the TBK Fat Loss Diet. For best results, add Wind Sprints and/or Walking 3 times a week.

1. Crossover Knee Raises

2. Jumping Jacks

3. Leg Pull-in/Extensions

4. Twisting Instep Touches

5. Forward Reaches

6. Burpees

7. Jumping Jacks

8. Crossover Knee Raises

9. Deep Knee Bends OR Floor Touches OR One-arm Floor Touches

10. Upper Body Sprints

Core Routine 7 – This is a routine for those of you who are at a higher fitness level.

1. Knuckle Push-ups OR Jackknife Push-ups OR Handstand Push-ups

2. Advanced Deep Knee Bends

3. Knuckle Push-ups OR Jackknife Push-ups OR Handstand Push-ups

4. Headstand Exercise

5. Knuckle Push-ups OR Jackknife Push-ups OR Handstand Push-ups

6. Front Kicks and/or Side Kicks

7. Knuckle Push-ups OR Jackknife Push-ups OR Handstand Push-ups

8. Wrestler's Bridge and/or Flat Bridge

9. Deep Breathing Exercises #1-3

Core Routine 8 – This routine will produce fantastic overall results by targeting all of your muscles from many different angles. In addition, it will add some variety to your workouts. This routine is performed slightly differently than the others in that you limit each exercise to as many as you can do in one minute before moving onto the next one. Thus the entire routine should take you approximately ½ hour to complete.

1. Underarm Touches

2. Deep Knee Bends

3. Side Arm Raises

4. Front Kicks

5. Overhead Arm Presses

6. Side Kicks

7. Rowing

8. Toe Touches

9. Arm Crossovers

10. Knee Raises

11. Arm Swings

12. Lunges

13. Forward Reaches

14. Knee Closing

15. Forward Bends

16. Neck Raises

17. Stationary Squat

18. Upper Body Sprints

19. Crossover Knee Raises

20. Push-ups OR Modified Push-ups

21. Neck Swings

22. Standing Push-ups

23. Calf Raises

24. Hand Walking Exercise

25. Twisting Instep Touches

26. Leg Pulls

27. Overhead Arm Raises

28. Bicycles

29. Alternate Punching

Core Routine 9 – This routine is for those of you involved in sports such as basketball, football, soccer, hockey, baseball, or tennis. **Remember to practice your sport specific skills.** Being in great shape won't compensate for lousy skills. In addition to the routine below, add some Wind Sprints and/or Squat Thrusts or Burpees 3 times a week.

1. Push-ups OR Knuckle Push-ups OR Jackknife Push-ups OR Handstand Push-ups

2. Deep Knee Bends OR Advanced Deep Knee Bends

3. Push-ups OR Knuckle Push-ups OR Jackknife Push-ups OR Handstand Push-ups

4. Crossover Knee Raises

5. Push-ups OR Knuckle Push-ups OR Jackknife Push-ups OR Handstand Push-ups

6. Floor Touches OR One-arm Floor Touches

7. Push-ups OR Knuckle Push-ups OR Jackknife Push-ups OR Handstand Push-ups

8. Leg Pull-in/Extensions

9. Twisting Instep Touches

10. Leg Pulls OR Leg Grasp

11. Front Kicks

12. Forward Bends

13. Neck Swings OR Resistance Neck Exercise OR Wrestler's Bridge

14. Deep Breathing Exercises #1-3

Core Routine 10 – This routine is for those of you involved in the grappling arts such as wrestling, judo, or ju-jitsu. **Remember not to neglect your grappling skills.** Add some Wind Sprints and/or Squat Thrusts or Burpees 3 times a week.

1. Push-ups OR Knuckle Push-ups OR Jackknife Push-ups OR Handstand Push-ups

2. Deep Knee Bends OR Advanced Deep Knee Bends

3. Push-ups OR Knuckle Push-ups OR Jackknife Push-ups OR Handstand Push-ups

4. Floor Touches OR One-arm Floor Touches

5. Push-ups OR Knuckle Push-ups OR Jackknife Push-ups OR Handstand Push-ups

6. Forward Bends

7. Push-ups OR Knuckle Push-ups OR Jackknife Push-ups OR Handstand Push-ups

8. Wrestler's Bridge

9. Side Kicks

10. Flat Bridge

11. Headstand Exercise

12. Leg Pulls OR Leg Grasp

13. Twisting Instep Touches

14. Deep Breathing Exercises #1-3

Core Routine 11 – Use this routine if you are involved in the striking arts such as boxing, karate, or tae kwondo. **Remember not to neglect your fighting skills.** Add Wind Sprints, shadow boxing, jumping rope, and/or bag work, and if involved in a kicking art add stretching as well. Try to break up the routine into 3 and a half minute rounds with a minute break in between to get into shape for a fight (A fight usually has three minute rounds, but the extra ½ minute will ensure that you are still running strong at the end of the round).

1. Push-ups OR Knuckle Push-ups OR Jackknife Push-ups OR Handstand Push-ups

2. Leg Pull-in/Extensions

3. Push-ups OR Knuckle Push-ups OR Jackknife Push-ups OR Handstand Push-ups

4. Leg Pull-in/Extensions

5. Push-ups OR Knuckle Push-ups OR Jackknife Push-ups OR Handstand Push-ups

6. Deep Knee Bends OR Advanced Deep Knee Bends

7. Push-ups OR Knuckle Push-ups OR Jackknife Push-ups OR Handstand Push-ups

8. Twisting Instep Touches

9. Front Kicks

10. Side Kicks

11. Neck Swings

12. Crossover Knee Raises

13. Forward Bends

14. Squat Thrusts OR Burpees

15. Flat Bridge

16. Deep Breathing Exercises #1-3

Core Routine 12 – The No Movement routine. Use this one for variety, or if you're trying to work out without making noise for people in the house or apartment building.

1. Cat Stretch

2. Stationary Squat

3. Leg Grasp

4. T-stance

5. Palm Press

6. Lower Back Press

7. Stomach Press

8. Wrestler's Bridge

9. Flat Bridge (optional)

Core Routine 13 – Punches and Kicks Routine. Use this one for variety and some fun once in a while. It's a great one for taking out your frustrations after a long day at the office ☺

1. Palm Strikes

2. Front Kicks

3. Alternate Punching

4. Side Kicks

5. Upper Cuts

6. Knee Raises

7. Neck Swings

Adding onto the Core Routines

In addition to the core routines, you may add any of the other exercises included in the program to your regimen, in order to strengthen a specific part of the body, to improve athleticism, or just to add some fun and variety to your workouts. You can add these additional exercises to the end of the core routine, or split things up, doing the core routine in the morning and the other exercises in the evening. If you are short on time, do the additional exercises only a few times a week, or on the weekends. Yet another strategy you can use is to do an exercise or two at odd moments during the day when you have a couple of free minutes. For example, you can do a set of push-ups and deep knee bends every hour that you're home. Certain exercises such as Stomach Presses, Lower Back Presses, Palm Presses, and some of the Deep Breathing Exercises can be done at the office without arousing too many odd looks. You can also go on a brisk walk during your lunch break.

Finally, it is a good idea to participate in physical activities which you enjoy. Although any of the core routines you follow will produce amazing results, being active in sports, martial arts, yoga, hiking, swimming, jumping rope, lifting weights, gardening, or just playing around with your children can make for a more rounded and interesting fitness program. The TBK Exercise Program will complement any type of physical activity or workout extremely well, ensuring excellent fitness.

Exercises

Advanced Deep Knee Bends

Advanced Deep Knee Bends work all of the muscles below the waist extremely well, and are an especially good leg exercise. When you can do 100-150 regular *Deep Knee Bends*, give these a try. Start in a standing position, hands on your hips, feet shoulder width apart or closer. Proceed to descend into a full squat, rising on your toes, until the back of your thighs touch your calves as shown to the right. Your trunk should remain fairly straight throughout the movement, although some slight forward bend is okay. Tighten your abdominal muscles on the way down to help keep your trunk straight. *Without bouncing or pausing at the bottom position*, proceed to return to the starting position by straightening out your legs. *As you ascend from the squat and straighten out your legs, shift most of your weight onto your right leg, but keep both feet on the floor.* Repeat, but this

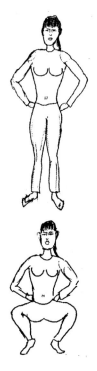

time, as you ascend, shift most of your weight onto your left leg. Repeat until tired, alternating legs. Inhale on the way up, exhale on the way down.

Alphabet Leg Raise

Leg Raises work the abs, hip flexors, lower back, and thighs. Start in a lying position, hands tucked underneath your lower back and butt. Raise your legs a few inches off of the floor, keeping your feet together and your legs straight as shown below. Pretend that you are holding a pen between your feet, and proceed to "write" the entire alphabet, from A to Z in the air, without letting your feet touch the ground. Breathe naturally during the performance of the exercise. For extra neck muscle work, keep your head off of the floor during the entire exercise.

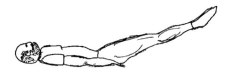

Alternate Punching

Alternate Punching works the muscles of the back, shoulders, and arms. Start in a standing position with your feet shoulder width apart, knees slightly bent, as shown below. Your hands should be placed close to your body, closed into fists, palm side up. Elbows should also be close to your body. Proceed to throw a straight punch with your left arm. As your arm moves out, it should simultaneously rotate such that when you finish the punch, your fist should be facing palm down. Do NOT fully lock out your elbow, rather, stop the punch just short of full extension. As soon as you complete the punch, rapidly pull your arm back to the starting position and repeat with the right arm. Continue until tired. Breathe naturally during this exercise. Aim for a pace of about 100-180 punches per minute.

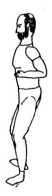
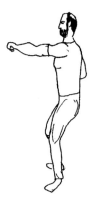

Arm Crossovers

Arm Crossovers work the muscles of the shoulders, chest, upper back, and arms. Start in a standing position, arms out and back as shown below. Proceed to rapidly bring the arms in front of the body, having them cross over each other, with the left one going over the right one, as shown below. Return to starting position, and repeat, this time having the right arm cross over the left. Continue until tired. Breathe naturally during this exercise. Aim for 60-100 crossovers per minute, but stay in control throughout the entire movement – do NOT jerk your arms back and forth, but instead move them smoothly.

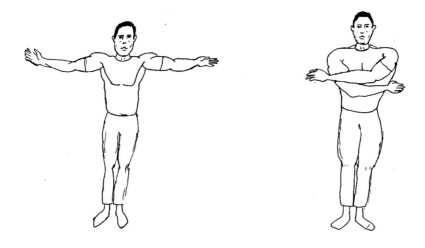

Arm Swings

Arm Swings work the muscles of the shoulders, back, and arms. Start in a standing position, legs about shoulder width apart, knees very slightly bent, arms out in front of the body at the level of the shoulders. Proceed to swing your arms all the way back while keeping your trunk straight. Without pausing, swing your arms back to the starting position. Repeat until tired. Breathe naturally throughout this movement. Aim for about 100-150 swings per minute. Stay in control, and use smooth, not jerky motions.

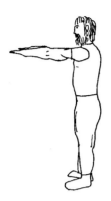 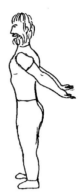

Bicycle

Bicycles work the muscles of the abs, hip flexors, lower back, and thighs. Start by lying on the floor on you back, with your hands tucked underneath your lower back and butt, legs up in the air with knees bent, as shown below. Pretend your feet are attached to bicycle pedals, and proceed to "ride" the bicycle until tired. Breathe naturally throughout the movement.

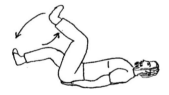

Burpee

The Burpee works pretty much all of the muscles in the body to some extent, and is a great exercise for losing weight as well as attaining cardiovascular fitness. Start by standing with your arms by your sides, feet about shoulder width apart. Proceed to squat down placing your hands on the floor on either side of your body. Next, keeping your hands where they are, with your arms straight, kick back into a push-up position by thrusting your legs back. This should be a smooth movement, with both of your legs moving and landing together. Next, hop with both feet from the push-up position back to the squat position, again keeping your hands and arms immobile. Finally stand up, returning to the starting position. Repeat until tired, but because this is a quite intense exercise, take it easy at the beginning. Breathe naturally throughout this movement. For extra intensity, instead of standing up during the last phase of the exercise, proceed to jump up as high as you can. In addition, you can also up the intensity by doing a push-up before returning to the squat position.

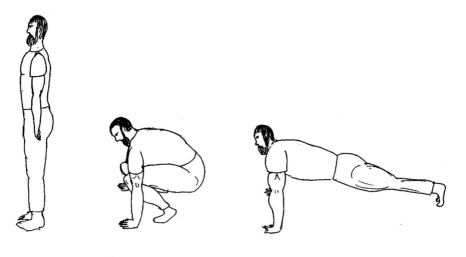

Calf Raise

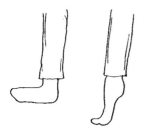

Calf Raises work the muscles of the calf, located in the back of the lower leg, as well as the muscles of the feet. From a standing position, feet about shoulder width apart, proceed to rise up onto your tip-toes. Return back to the starting position, and repeat until tired. Breathe naturally during this movement. For added intensity, perform one legged calf raises. Start by standing on one foot, holding a sturdy chair for balance if desired, and proceed to rise up onto your tiptoes. Repeat until tired, and then repeat with the other foot.

Cat Stretch

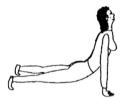

The Cat Stretch works the muscles of the arms, chest, shoulders, and back, as well as improves flexibility. The exercise consists of holding the position below until tired. Your arms are straight and slightly wider than shoulder width apart. Your legs are straight and wider than shoulder width apart. Your entire body is supported by your hands and tiptoes – no other part should be touching the floor (although your legs will be very close to the floor). Your head should be looking up. Breathe naturally while holding the cat stretch.

Crossover Knee Raise

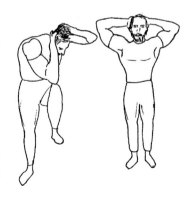

Crossover knee raises work the muscles of the waist, hip flexors, and thighs. Start in a standing position with your hands clasped behind your head. Proceed to touch your left knee with your right elbow as shown to the right. Return to the starting position, and proceed to touch your right knee with your left elbow. Return to the starting position and repeat until tired. Breathe naturally while performing this exercise.

Deep Breathing Exercises

Deep Breathing Exercises are an underused, yet beneficial way of developing the body and improving health. These exercises develop lung power, reduce stress, and depending on which exercise you are doing, work various other muscles. Deep breathing is best done outside in fresh air. Do these exercises several times during the day at odd moments, as well as at night in bed.

Deep Breathing Exercise #1

Take a very deep breath through your mouth and nose, completely filling up your lungs. Now hold it for 10-20 seconds, and exhale, forcing every last bit of air out. Take a few regular breaths, and repeat 5-10 times.

Deep Breathing Exercise #2

Take a very deep breath through your mouth, completely filling up your lungs. Hold it for a second, and exhale forcefully, expelling the air out of your lungs as fast as possible. Take a few normal breaths, and repeat 5-10 times.

Deep Breathing Exercise #3

Start in a standing position, arms hanging freely at your sides, elbows slightly bent, feet shoulder width apart. Proceed to slowly take a deep breath, completely filling up your lungs. Exhale slowly. *After*

you finish exhaling, and before taking the next breath, tense your chest muscles for 2 seconds. Repeat once more. Next, take another deep breath, and this time, after exhaling, tense your arm muscles (without moving your arm). Repeat once again. Next, repeat twice, but this time tensing your latissimus dorsi muscles (these are the large, wing-like muscles of the middle back). After that, repeat with your abs, then twice with your thigh muscles. Finish off with a few deep breaths without contracting anything.

Deep Breathing Exercise # 4

This looks quite similar to the arm crossovers, but it is a different exercise. Start in a standing position, arms out to the sides as shown. Take a deep breath, and as you exhale, slowly move your arms across 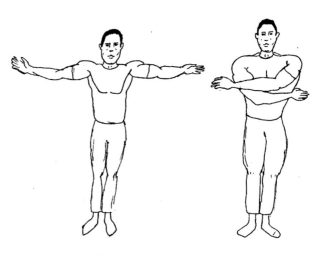 the body as shown, and finish off the movement by squeezing your chest muscles. Inhale, slowly bring the arms back to the starting position, and repeat, but this time whichever arm was on the bottom during the final part of the movement should be on top. Repeat 5-10 times.

Deep Knee Bend

Deep Knee Bends are one of the best leg exercises, and work most of the rest of the muscles below the waist. In addition, they provide an excellent cardiovascular workout. To do a deep knee bend, start in a standing position, feet shoulder width apart or closer, toes slightly turned out, hands hanging freely at your sides. Proceed to squat all the way down, rising on your toes, until the back of your thighs touch your calves as shown below. As you go down, let your arms

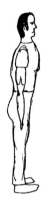
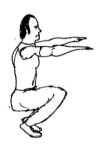

swing forward for balance. Your trunk should remain fairly straight throughout the movement, although some slight forward bend is okay. Tighten your abdominal muscles on the way down to help keep your trunk straight. ***Without pausing or bouncing at the bottom position***, straighten your legs, returning to the starting position. Repeat until tired. Exhale on the way down, inhale on the way up. If you need to, hold onto a sturdy piece of furniture for balance, but eventually try to do these without assistance, as doing so will yield superior results. Aim for a pace of 20-40 a minute.

Flat Bridge

The flat bridge is a very intense exercise that works the neck, abs, lower back and legs. Use caution when performing it. Perform this exercise on your bed, or use a mat or some other padded surface to place your forehead on. The entire exercise consists of getting into the position shown below, in which your entire body is completely straight and is resting entirely on your forehead and toes, and holding this position until tired. Breathe naturally during this movement.

107

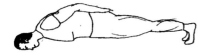

Floor Touch

Floor Touches target the muscles of the legs, trunk, and lower back. They also yield cardiovascular benefits. Start in a standing position, arms hanging at your sides. Keeping your feet flat on the floor, proceed to squat down and touch the floor in front of your feet as shown below. Stand back up. Repeat until tired. Inhale on the way up, exhale on the way down. Aim for a pace of 30 or so a minute.

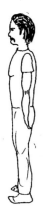
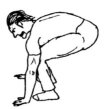

Forward Bend

Forward Bends work the muscles of the back, trunk, hamstrings, butt, shoulders, and triceps. Start in a standing position with your arms out in front of your body at the level of your shoulders. Proceed to bend forward at the waist, simultaneously bending your knees a bit and swinging your arms all the way back as far as they will go, as shown below. Return to the starting position and repeat until your muscles feel moderately fatigued. Inhale on the way up, exhale while bending. Aim for a pace of 20-30 a minute.

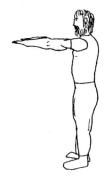

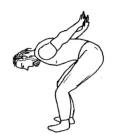

Forward Reach

Forward Reaches work the muscles of the abs and shoulders. Start in a standing position, hands clenched into fists resting on your chest. Keeping your back straight, proceed to lean forward while simultaneously extending your arms out. Return to the starting position and repeat until tired. Exhale while extending your arms, inhale while returning them to your body. Aim for a pace of about 20 a minute.

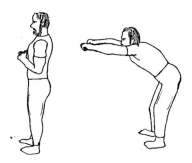

Front Kick

Front Kicks work the muscles of the abs, hip flexor, and thighs, as well as improve flexibility. Starting from a standing position, proceed to kick your left leg forward as high as it will comfortably go without straining. Return to the starting position, and repeat until tired. Next, repeat with the right leg. Breathe naturally during the performance of this exercise. Aim for a pace of 30-40 kicks per minute.

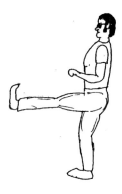

Handstand Push-up

Handstand Push-ups work nearly every single muscle above the waist extremely well, and to some extent provide a workout for the entire body. They are probably the single best exercise for building upper-body muscle mass. *Use extreme caution when performing a handstand as it is quite advanced. Do NOT perform this exercise if you suffer from high blood pressure.* Facing a sturdy wall (*WITHOUT a window*), place your hands a few inches from the wall, slightly wider than shoulder width apart, and proceed to kick up into a handstand, resting your feet against the wall for balance as shown below. When you have steadied yourself, Keep your head up, and *carefully* proceed to dip down until the top of your forehead *lightly* touches the floor. Press yourself back up, and repeat until tired. Inhale while lowering yourself, exhale while pushing back up. A different exercise you can do is to simply hold the handstand position for as long as you can, breathing naturally.

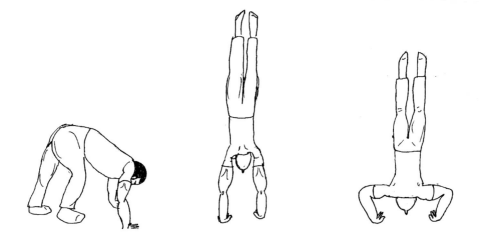

Hand Walking Exercise

The Hand Walking Exercise works the muscles of the triceps, back, abs, and chest. Start on your hands and knees, knees resting on a towel or mat, back straight, hands shoulder width apart. Proceed to walk your hands away from your body

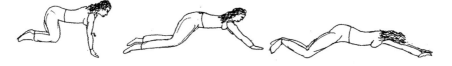

until they can go no further. Keep your knees on the floor. Towards the end, your feet will come up off of the floor. That's okay, as long as your knees remain in place. Walk your hands back to the starting position and repeat until tired. Breathe naturally during this exercise.

Headstand Exercise

The Headstand Exercise works the muscles of the neck, spine, trunk, and to some extent most of the rest of the muscles of the body. ***Do NOT perform this exercise if you suffer from high blood pressure.*** Before beginning, place a mat or folded towel on the floor where your head will go. Kneel down on the floor facing a sturdy wall (***WITHOUT a window***). You won't actually be using the wall during the exercise, but in case you lose your balance it will prevent you from falling backwards and injuring yourself. Place your hands on the floor in front of you spaced wider than shoulder width apart. Place your head on the floor in front of your hands (closer to the wall), such that your head and hands form a triangle, as shown below. Proceed to put your right knee on your right elbow and your left knee on your left elbow. Slowly straighten your legs out over your head. At this point you have completed the headstand. You can do a number of different exercises now. The first is just holding the headstand for a minute or so. The second consists of opening and closing your legs like scissors. The last and most challenging exercise is to bring your knees to your chest and then back up again until tired. Breathe naturally during the performance of this exercise, taking care NOT to hold your breath.

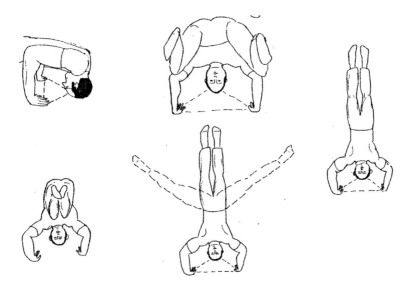

Jackknife Push-up

The Jackknife Push-up is an excellent upper body exercise, working the muscles of the shoulders, chest, arms, and back. It is a hybrid exercise between a standard push-up and a handstand push-up. Start in the position shown below to the left, hands slightly wider than shoulder width apart, feet much wider than shoulder width apart, butt up in the air, legs and back straight, arms straight, chin tucked into your chest. Proceed to *carefully* dip down by bending your arms until the top of your head *lightly* touches the floor. Your arms are the only part of the body that should be moving. Push back up and repeat until tired. Inhale on the way down, exhale when pushing up.

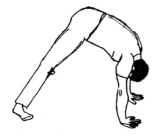 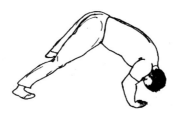

Jumping Jacks

Jumping Jacks work the muscles of the legs, shoulders, and arms, and are excellent for cardiovascular fitness and weight loss. Start in a standing position, feet together, arms hanging at the sides as shown below. Proceed to jump up a couple of inches, simultaneously spreading your legs and raising your arms in a semi-circular motion above your head as shown by the dotted lines. Jump again, returning to the starting position, and repeat until tired. Breathe naturally during the performance of this exercise.

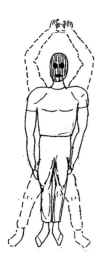

Knee Closing

Knee Closing works the muscles of the chest, arms, and the outer thighs. Start in a standing position, feet about shoulder width apart, trunk hunched over with your hands on the outside of your knees as shown below. Proceed to force your knees together, resisting the entire way with your outer thighs. As soon as your knees touch, open

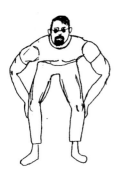 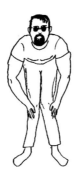

your knees again and repeat until tired. Breathe naturally during this exercise, taking care NOT to hold your breath.

Knee Raise

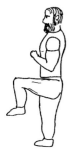

Knee Raises work the muscles of the abs, hip flexors, and thighs. Start in a standing position, hands by your chest or hanging at your sides. Proceed to raise your left thigh to about waist level (or higher), and lower it back down to starting position. Repeat until tired. Next, repeat with your right leg. Breathe naturally while performing this exercise.

Knuckle Push-up

Knuckle Push-ups work the muscles of the chest, arms, shoulders, and back, in addition to most of the other muscles of the body to some extent. This exercise is done in the exact same way as a normal push-up, so look up *Push-up* for instructions on how to perform one. The only difference is that a knuckle push-up is performed on closed fists as shown below.

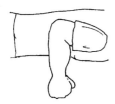

Land Swimming

Land Swimming works the muscles of the spine, shoulders, butt, and the back of the thighs. Start by lying down on your stomach with your arms extended out straight above your head and your legs straight. Keeping your leg straight, proceed to raise your left leg and right arm simultaneously off of the floor. Return to the starting position, and repeat with your right leg and left arm. Continue until tired. Breathe naturally when performing this exercise.

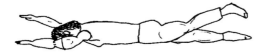

Leg Grasp

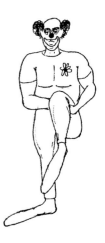

Leg Grasps work the muscles of the biceps, back, and forearms. The entire exercise consists of holding the position shown to the right, in which you clasp your hands underneath your knee, and pull up the knee as far as it will go towards the chest. Hold the knee at that top position for as long as you can, breathing naturally and taking care NOT to hold your breath. Release the leg, shake your arms and rest for a little while, and repeat the exercise with the other leg.

Leg Pull

Leg Pulls work the biceps, upper back, and the grip muscles, as well as improve balance. Start by grasping the back of your left thigh above the knee with your left hand, as shown to the right. Proceed to pull the left leg up and back as far as possible. Return to the starting position ***without*** letting your left foot touch the floor. Continue until tired. Repeat with the right arm and leg. Breathe naturally while performing this exercise.

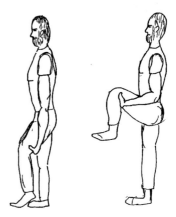

Leg Pull-in/Extension.

Leg Pull-in/extensions work the muscles of your abs, hips, and lower back. Start by lying flat on the floor, hands tucked underneath your lower back/butt as shown below. Proceed to pull your legs into your chest. Next, extend your legs above your head. Lower them back down to the middle position, and push them out straight to the first position, but without letting your feet touch the floor. Repeat until tired. Breathe naturally throughout the exercise.

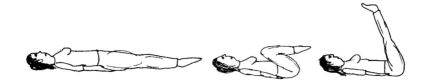

Lower Back Press

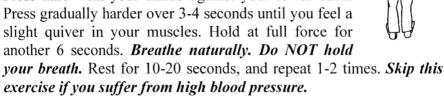

The Lower Back Press works the muscles of the chest, back, shoulders, and arms. In a standing position, place both hands palms flat against your lower back. Press hard with your hands against your lower back. Press gradually harder over 3-4 seconds until you feel a slight quiver in your muscles. Hold at full force for another 6 seconds. ***Breathe naturally. Do NOT hold your breath.*** Rest for 10-20 seconds, and repeat 1-2 times. ***Skip this exercise if you suffer from high blood pressure.***

Lunge

Lunges work the muscles of the thigh. Start in a standing position, with your right leg in front of your body and your left leg behind your body. Both legs should be straight. Proceed to dip down by bending your right knee until your left knee *lightly* touches the floor. Your right foot should not move at all. Your left foot will come off the floor onto its tiptoes, but otherwise should not move. Return to the starting position. Continue until tired and then repeat with the left foot. Inhale on the way down, exhale on the way up.

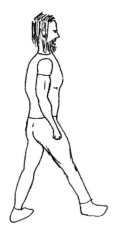
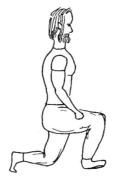

Lying Shoulder Exercise

The Lying Shoulder Exercise works the muscles of... yep... you guessed it, the shoulders. Lie down on the floor on your stomach, arms at your sides, a couple of inches off of the floor, palms down. Proceed to move both arms simultaneously in a semicircle until they reach a position stretched out in front of your body, as shown by the dotted lines. Return to the starting position and repeat until tired. Breathe naturally during this exercise, and aim for a pace of 20 per minute.

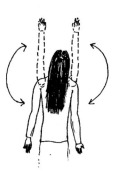

Modified Push-ups

Modified Push-ups work the muscles of the chest, arms, and shoulders. To do a Modified Push-up, start in the position shown below, knees on floor, hands on the floor slightly wider than shoulder width apart, back straight. Proceed to bend your elbows, bringing your upper body towards the floor until your chin lightly touches the floor. Without pausing or bouncing, proceed to straighten your arms, returning to the starting position. Inhale when lowering, exhale when pushing up. When you can do 50 or more Modified Push-ups, switch to regular Push-ups.

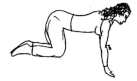
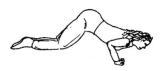

Neck Raise

Neck Raises work the muscles of the neck. This is a two part movement. Start off by lying on your stomach, arms at your sides. Proceed to raise your head up off of the floor. Lower it back down, and repeat until tired. For the next part of the movement, roll over onto your back, and proceed to once again raise your head off of the floor until your chin touches the top of your chest. Continue until tired. Breathe naturally while performing this exercise.

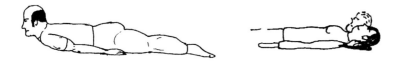

Neck Swing

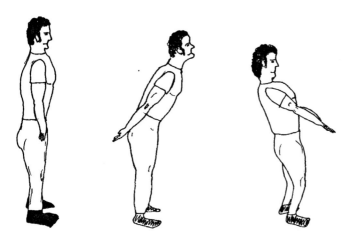

Neck Swings work the muscles of the neck. Start in a standing position, arms hanging at your sides. Proceed to lean forward, extending your head out as you lean. Without pausing, proceed to change directions and lean back. On the way back, tuck your chin towards the back of your neck, as shown below. Continue until tired. ***This should be a smooth, gentle, continuous motion, not jerky.*** Start out slowly, and when your neck muscles are somewhat looser and warmed up, you can up the tempo a bit up to a pace of 40-60 per minute. Breathe naturally while performing this exercise, and let your arms swing freely.

One-arm Floor Touch

One-arm Floor Touches target the muscles of the legs, trunk, and lower back. They also yield cardiovascular benefits. Start in a standing position, arms hanging at your sides. Keeping your feet flat on the floor, proceed to squat down and touch the floor in front of your feet with your right hand, simultaneously bringing your left arm behind your back as shown below. Stand back up. Repeat with your left arm. Continue until tired. Inhale on the way up, exhale on the way down. Aim for a pace of 30 or so a minute.

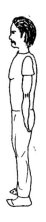
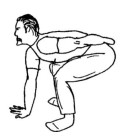

One-arm Standing Push-up

One-arm Standing Push-ups work the muscles of the arm, shoulder, and chest. Start in the position shown below, with your right leg out in front of your body, right knee slightly bent, left leg back and straight, left arm hanging freely. Brace your right hand above your right knee. Proceed to fully bend your right arm, lowering your upper body. Next, ***using only your arm and chest muscles, NOT your trunk or lower back***, push back up to the starting position. Continue until tired, then do the exercise with your left hand on your left knee. Inhale on the way down, exhale on the way up. Aim for a pace of 30 or so per minute.

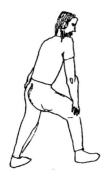 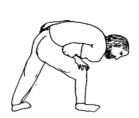

One Minute Push-up

The One Minute Push-up works the muscles of the upper body extremely well, and to some extent works most of the muscles in the body. Start in the position shown below, feet together, hands slightly wider than shoulder width apart, back and legs straight and in line with each other. Keeping your back and legs straight, proceed to bend your elbows, lowering yourself about a quarter of the way down towards the floor. Hold this position for a slow count of 15. Next, bend your elbows even more, going down to about half way towards the floor, and hold for another slow count of 15. Now bend your elbows even more, such that your chest is almost touching the floor, and hold for another slow count of 15. Finally, return to the starting position, and hold for a final count of 15. Breathe naturally during the exercise, making sure NOT to hold your breath.

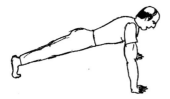

Overhead Arm Raise

The Overhead Arm Raise works the front part of the shoulder muscle. Start in a standing position, arms resting in front of the body, right hand resting on top of the left hand, holding on. Keeping the right hand on top of the left, lift the left arm straight up and over your body. Do not resist with the right hand, but keep it on top of the left the entire time. Lower the left arm back down, and continue until tired. Repeat with the left hand resting on the right. Inhale on the way up, exhale on the way down. Aim for a pace of 30 or so raises a minute.

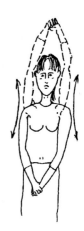

Overhead Arm Press

The Overhead Arm Press works the muscles of the shoulders and arm. Start in a standing position right arm bent with right hand clenched into a fist, left hand resting on it lightly holding on. Keeping your left hand on your right, proceed to press your right hand up and over your head as shown. Do not resist with the left hand, but keep it on top of the right the entire time. Lower the arm back to the starting position, and continue until tired. Repeat with the right hand resting on the left. Breathe naturally during this movement, and aim for a pace of 30 or so presses a minute.

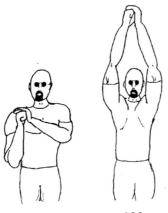

Palm Press

The Palm Press works the muscles of the chest, arms, shoulders, and hands. Start in a standing or sitting position with your palms together flat against each other. Press hard with your hands against each other. Press gradually harder over 3-4 seconds until you feel a slight quiver in your muscles. Hold at full force for another 6 seconds. ***Breathe naturally. Do NOT hold your breath.*** Rest for 10-20 seconds, and repeat 1-2 times. ***Skip this exercise if you suffer from high blood pressure.***

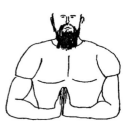

Palm Strikes

Palm Strikes work the muscles of the arms, shoulders, chest, back, trunk, and hips. Start in a standing position, left leg in front of the right, arms up at chest level, hands open. Proceed to strike with your left arm, extending it front of your body (but without locking the elbow). Next, retract your left arm, simultaneously throwing a palm strike with your right arm. Retract your right arm, and throw an elbow with your left arm as shown below. Repeat the entire sequence 5 times. Then proceed to shift your legs such that the right leg is in front, and repeat the entire sequence 5 times, but this time throwing the first strike with the right arm. Continue switching back and forth until tired. When throwing the strikes and elbows, use your hips and your body. A strike or elbow initiates in the feet. Look at the third drawing from the left carefully. Notice how the foot turns and goes up to the tiptoes, transferring the power through the leg, hip, trunk, shoulder, and into the arm. Breathe naturally during this exercise.

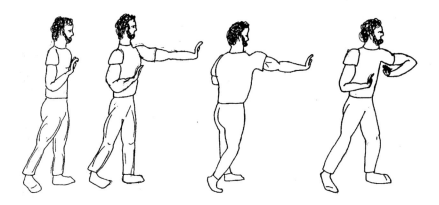

Pelvic Lift

The Pelvic Lift works the muscles of the lower back, butt, hamstrings, and abs. Lie on your back with your knees bent, feet flat on the floor and together, arms lying at your sides. Proceed to lift your butt off of the floor while keeping your feet flat. Pause at the top for a second, and return to the starting position. Repeat until tired. Breathe naturally during this exercise.

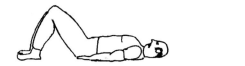 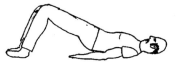

Push-ups

Push-ups work the upper body muscles extremely well, and in addition work many of the other muscles of the body to some extent. If you cannot do at least 5-10 push-ups, substitute *Modified Push-ups* or *Standing Push-ups* instead. To do a push-up, start in the position shown below, feet together, hands slightly wider than shoulder width apart, back and legs straight and in line with each other, head up. Keeping your back and legs straight, proceed to bend your elbows,

125

lowering your body until your chest lightly touches the floor. Without pausing or bouncing, straighten your arms, returning to the starting position. Repeat until tired. Inhale when lowering your body, exhale when pushing up. Aim for a pace of 30 or so push-ups per minute.

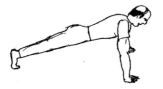 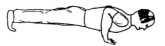

Resistance Neck Exercise

The Resistance Neck Exercise works all of the muscles of the neck. It is a six part exercise. Start by clasping your hands over your forehead. Proceed to touch your chin to your chest, resisting with firm but gentle pressure from your hands the entire way down. Now, using your hands, firmly but gently force your head back, resisting with your neck muscles the entire way. Repeat until tired. Next, clasp your hands behind your head, and firmly but gently force your head towards your chest, resisting with your neck muscles the entire way. As soon as your chin touches your chest, reverse the movement, forcing your head back while offering resistance with your hands. Continue until tired. Next, put your right hand against the right side of your head and repeat the exercise from side to side. Repeat using the left hand. Finally, with your hand against the side of your head, turn your head to the side, again using both the right and left hands. Breathe naturally while performing the exercise taking care NOT to hold your breath. Aim for a pace of about 15 per minute.

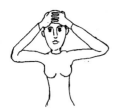 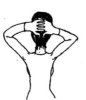 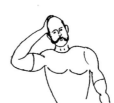 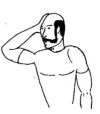

Rowing

Rowing works the muscles of the arms, shoulders, and back. Start in a standing position with your arms extended out straight in front of your body. Proceed to pull them in towards your body. Return to the starting position and continue until tired. Breathe naturally while performing this exercise. Aim for a pace of 30-60 rows per minute.

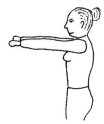 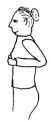

Running in Place

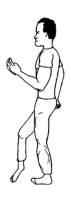

Running in place works the muscles of the thighs, hip flexors, calves, and provides a cardiovascular workout. To perform this exercise, simply run in place. Change the intensity, running slow some of the time, and fast at others. Another way to increase the intensity is to lift your knees up higher. Breathe naturally during your run.

Side Arm Raise

Side Arm Raises work the muscles of the shoulder. Start in a standing position, hands lying by your stomach. Grasp your left hand with your right and lift your right elbow up and to the side of the body, as shown below. Do not resist with the left arm. Lower it back down to the starting position, and repeat until tired. Next, repeat with the left hand holding the right. Breathe naturally during this exercise. Aim for a pace of about 30 or so raises a minute.

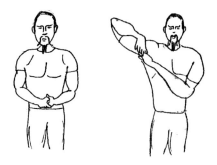

Side Kick

Side Kicks work the muscles located at the side of the trunk (obliques), the outer portion of the thighs, and the hip flexors, as well as improve flexibility. Start in a standing position holding your hands together in front of your body or up by your chest. Proceed to kick your left leg out to the side of your body as high as it will comfortably go. Continue kicking until tired, and then repeat the exercise with your right leg. Breathe naturally during this exercise, and only kick as high as you can without straining. Aim for a pace of 30-40 kicks per minute.

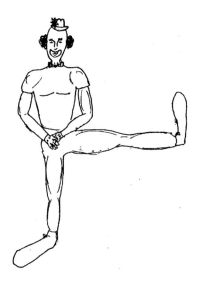

Squat Thrust

Squat Thrusts work most of the muscles of the body, and are great for weight loss as well as cardiovascular fitness. Start in a squat with your hands on the floor on either side of your body, as shown below. Next, keeping your hands where they are, with your arms straight, kick back into a push-up position by thrusting your legs back. This should be a smooth movement, with both of your legs moving and landing together. Next, hop with both feet from the push-up position back to the squat position, again keeping your hands and arms immobile. Continue until tired. This is quite an intense exercise, so take it easy at first. Breathe naturally during this exercise.

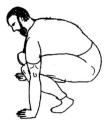 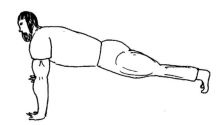

Standing Push-up

Standing Push-ups work the muscles of the arms, chest, and shoulders. Start in a standing position, hunched over with your hands braced above your knees, which should be slightly bent. Your feet should be about shoulder width apart. Proceed to lower your upper body as far down 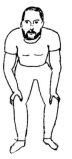 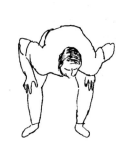 as possible by bending your arms. Next, *using only your arm and chest muscles, NOT your trunk or lower back,* push back up to the starting position. Continue until tired. Inhale on the way down, exhale on the way up. Aim for a pace of about 30 push-ups per minute. When you can do 50 or more Standing Push-ups, switch to regular push-ups.

Stationary Squat

The Stationary Squat works the muscles of the legs. Start in a standing position, feet spaced wider than shoulder width apart, toes slightly turned out, and proceed to descend into a squat until your thighs are parallel to the floor. Keep your feet flat on the floor and try to "grip" the floor with your toes. Extend both of your arms out in front of your body, and hold this position until tired. Breathe naturally – do NOT hold your breath.

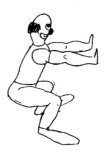

Stomach Press

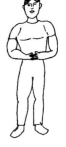

The Stomach Press works the muscles of the chest, shoulders, back, and arms. Clasp both hands over your stomach. Press hard with your hands against your stomach. Press gradually harder over 3-4 seconds until you feel a slight quiver in your muscles. Hold at full force for another 6 seconds. ***Breathe naturally. Do NOT hold your breath.*** Rest for 10-20 seconds, and repeat 1-2 times. ***Skip this exercise if you suffer from high blood pressure.***

Swing Thru

Swing Thrus work the muscles of the spine, butt, thighs, abs, shoulders, and are excellent for cardiovascular fitness and weight loss. Start in a standing position, hands over your head, lightly clasped together, feet slightly wider than shoulder width apart, toes slightly out. Proceed to swing your hands through your legs as far back as possible, bending your knees on the way down, as shown below. Return to the starting position, using your butt and hamstring muscles to assist your lower back. Repeat until moderately fatigued. Inhale on the way up, exhale on the way down. Aim for a pace of 20-30 swings per minute.

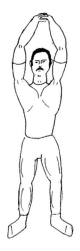

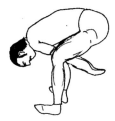

Toe Touches

Toe touches work the muscles of the spine, trunk, butt, and the back of the thighs (hamstrings), as well as improve flexibility. To do a toe touch, start in the position shown below, feet shoulder width apart, legs straight, hands extended overhead, trunk slightly leaning back. Keeping your legs straight, bend forward and touch your toes or the floor in front of your toes (if you can't touch your toes, go down as far as you can without straining, and gradually try to improve your reach). *As you go down, tighten your abdominal muscles.* Proceed to return your body to the starting position, *using the muscles of your butt and hamstrings* to assist your back muscles. Repeat until moderately fatigued. Inhale on the way up, exhale on the way down.

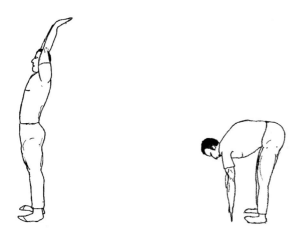

T-stance

The T-stance works the muscles of the spine, trunk, abs, leg, and shoulders, as well as develops balance and flexibility. Start in a standing position with your hands stretched up above your head. Proceed to bend forward, simultaneously raising your right leg backwards until your body forms a "T" as shown below. Keep a slight bend in your knee. Hold this position for a minute or more, and repeat with your left leg. Breathe naturally during this exercise.

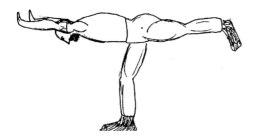

Twisting Instep Touch

Twisting Instep Touches work the entire musculature of the trunk, including the abs, lower back, and obliques, as well as the muscles of the butt and the back of the thighs (hamstrings). In addition, they improve flexibility. Start in a standing position, feet spaced shoulder width apart (or closer or wider, whichever is your preference), arms out at shoulder level. Proceed to bend to the left side, raising your right arm over your head while simultaneously touching your right instep with your left hand as shown below. Reverse the motion back to the starting position, and proceed to bend to your right, raising your left arm over your head while touching your left instep with your right hand. Reverse the motion back to the starting position and continue until moderately tired, but NOT to the point where you cannot do anymore. Inhale on the way up, exhale on the way down.

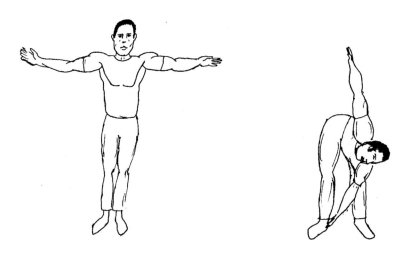

Underarm Touch

Underarm touches work the muscles of the shoulders, upper back, and arms. Start in a standing position with your hands at your sides. Proceed to rapidly raise both hands simultaneously up along side the body until they touch your underarms. Keep your elbows high during the movement. Continue until tired. Breathe naturally during this exercise. Aim for a pace of 50-75 touches per minute.

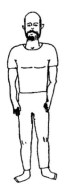 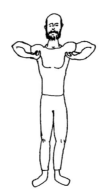

Upper Body Sprints

Upper Body Sprints work most of the muscles of the upper body, and are great for cardiovascular fitness and for burning fat. Start in a standing position with your feet together, and proceed to sprint as fast as you can, using only your arms and upper body, *without* moving your legs or feet, which stay planted flat on the floor throughout the exercise. In essence, you are doing only the upper body part of a regular sprint. Continue until tired. Rest for 20-30 seconds, and repeat 3-5 more times. Breathe naturally during this exercise, taking care NOT to hold your breath.

Uppercuts

Uppercuts work the muscles of the hips, trunk, back, chest, shoulders, and arms. Start in a standing position, feet about shoulder width apart, arms bent and fists clenched at about chest level. Proceed to throw an uppercut with your right arm as shown to the right. Your arm should not bend or extend at all during the movement. Study the picture

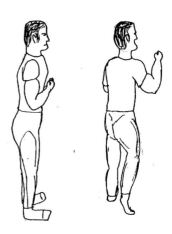

carefully. The movement originates in the feet. Pivot your foot, slightly flexing your hip as the power of the punch is transferred through the hips, which turn, through the trunk, chest, and into the shoulder and arm. Lower your right arm, and simultaneously throw an uppercut with your left arm. Continue until tired. Breathe naturally while performing this exercise.

Walking

Walking is a great exercise for people of all fitness levels. If done properly, it provides a good workout for many of the muscles below the waist, especially those of the lower legs, as well as enhances cardiovascular fitness. Ideally, you should walk in nature, and avoid polluted areas such as cities. Hiking outdoors, especially on hilly or mountainous terrain, can be challenging even to people in good shape. Walk at a brisk pace, swinging your arms and breathing naturally.

Wind Sprints

Wind Sprints work practically every muscle in the body, especially those of the legs, and enhance speed and cardiovascular fitness, making them one of the best all around exercise in existence. Begin by warming up through a few minutes of brisk walking. Proceed to sprint as fast as you can for 10-30 seconds. Slow down and walk for 30-60 seconds, and do another sprint. Repeat this cycle until tired. ***Do NOT overdo this exercise initially.*** Start with 2 or so sprints, and slowly build up. For added intensity, do hill sprints. Sprint up a hill, walk down, and repeat. Alternatively, do a set of push-ups after each sprint.

Wrestler's Bridge

The Wrestler's Bridge is an excellent exercise that targets the muscles of the neck, upper back, spine, trunk, hips, and legs. Perform this exercise on your bed, or place your head on a mat or some other padded surface. Start by lying on your back, knees bent, feet flat and shoulder width apart. Proceed to ***slowly and carefully*** roll your head back such that you end up in the position shown below, where the entire weight of your body is resting on your head and feet and your arms are folded over your chest. Hold this position until tired. Breathe naturally while performing the bridge. ***Do NOT perform this exercise if you suffer from high blood pressure.***

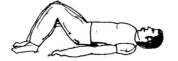 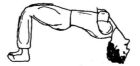

Exercises You Should Avoid

In this last segment I will discuss some types of exercise which are better left alone. The first is jogging. Jogging at a moderate intensity, especially for long periods of time and on a level, hard surface, will most likely lead to a repetitive strain injury of the knees, ankles, and/or hips. It is much better to do Wind Sprints interspersed with fast walking or if you want, jogging. The high intensity sprints will tire you out faster, cutting the duration of the jog and thus saving your joints. It is also better to run on surfaces such as grass or sand, or to run hills rather than to jog on asphalt or concrete. Other types of long duration, medium to low intensity repetitive type exercise should be avoided as well. This includes the step machines, ski machines, and exercise bicycles, in which you perform the same movement along the same track thousands of times.

Avoid ab machines, as they are a useless, expensive waste of money. First of all, to have well defined abs, you need to shed that layer of fat around them. Second, doing crunch type exercises gives you very little functional strength, since in life, muscle groups are rarely if ever used in isolation. Isolating the abs makes you good at doing ab machine crunches. That's it. The same goes for most exercise machines as well, which tend to isolate single muscles. You're better off spending your time on more useful exercises.

Tamir B. Katz, M.D.

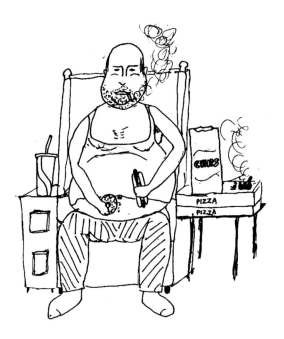

Part 3 – Why Diet, Exercise, & Smoking Cessation Programs Fail And What You Can Do About It

In this section, I will be discussing why our fitness programs fail, and what to do about it. After all, what good is the best program if you are not going to stick to it. I'll start off with a typical scenario. It's New Year's Eve. You pat your gut, or look at your expanding hips that no longer fit into the skirt that you bought just last year. Then you make your New Year's resolution. You know the one. It goes something like "I'll lose so and so pounds or inches off of my waist." And you mean it. You tell your significant other about the diet that you are starting tomorrow and the gym that you have just joined. For the next few weeks, you actually stick to it. Just like last year. Just like every other year. You suffer when going out to dinner with your family. While they are enjoying the all-you-can-eat buffet, you look at the measly salad on your plate. When dessert comes, you look wide eyed at everyone else's triple fudge chocolate cake and hope that someone offers you a small bite. Day after day, you stop by the gym on the way home from work, sweating away on the treadmill, pumping those weights. But then, day after day becomes every other day. At work, you sneak in half a donut with your cup of coffee in the morning. Within a month, a half a donut becomes at least 2 donuts, and you find yourself leading the way to the all you can eat buffet, mouth watering, with two large plates in your hands. The gym becomes a vague memory of drenching sweat, hard work and too many people in spandex.

You can't figure out how it happens. It just does. The first few times you skip a workout or cheat on your diet, there are probably legitimate reasons. You were working late at the office, so you joined in when the pizza or takeout arrived. You had to catch your kid's school play, so you skipped that workout at the gym. Etc. Etc. But in hindsight, as time went on, the reasons for skipping the gym or going off of your diet became lamer and lamer, until you yourself could no longer rationalize any of them. I can run through a similar scenario with quitting smoking, or any other matter of compliance, such as taking your blood pressure medications as prescribed.

Why *do* we fail? Is it because we are weak? Is it because we just don't care enough? Is it simply not worth it? Is the program too strict? Or is it because we simply don't have the social support or environment to effect a major lifestyle change? There is no one right answer. Below, I hope to simply outline and discuss my suggestions on successfully implementing a diet, exercise, and smoking cessation program.

Before we delve into how to stick to a program, I think the million dollar question that has to be asked is, **"Is it worth it?"** The answer to that question is different for different people. Let's lay out the facts on the table. If you live a healthy life, meaning you eat right, exercise, don't smoke or drink too much, and cut down on your stress levels, you will probably live to an older age. However, we are probably talking about up to no more than 10 extra years, and leading a healthy life is no guarantee you'll live to be over a 100 years old (you need good genes for that). **However, more importantly, your *quality* of life will improve.** What I mean by that is that when you hit 80, instead of vegetating in a wheelchair, short of breath, full of aches and pains, you'll be playing tag with your grandchildren. Nowadays, with all of the advancements in medicine, even sickly people often live a long time. People can live with a damaged heart for years. However, during those years, they are not too active, they have to be on many medications, and they probably end up in the hospital many times, undergoing multiple procedures and operations with all of the associated pain, discomfort, and complications. Thus, logically, getting into shape seems like a worthwhile investment. But again, although that seems logical *to me*, to some people, "living the good life" – eating plenty of any food they wish, smoking, drinking, not exercising, is more worth it than a few more years. That's their prerogative.

Another thing to consider is how much are you willing to invest, or **how much is it worth it?** Perhaps you are willing to do a few minutes of exercise a day, but no more. Or maybe you are willing to eat less junk food, smoke fewer cigarettes, or have one less beer with dinner. The point I'm making here is that life isn't black and white. You don't have to either live a spartan life, waking up at dawn for 3 hours of calisthenics and a five mile hike, eating grasses and roots, or on the other extreme having donuts for breakfast, burgers, fries, and soda for lunch, and pizza and ice cream for dinner. Fitness is a spectrum, and each of you has to decide how much you are willing to do.

This is why diets tend to fail. **Each of you has to find a fitness plan that you can stick to *for life*.** There is a role for diets and marathon exercise programs, such as when you are trying to quickly lose a few pounds for a wedding or a high school reunion, but you'll quickly gain the weight back when you return to your old diet. This is a crucial point. **You have to decide what *permanent* changes you want to include in your life.** I have tried to think about that in my fitness program. The basic program takes only minutes a day. The diet is pretty strict, but I did include a less strict diet of several foods to exclude, which, when combined with the exercise program, can yield very good results. Alternatively, you can do what I do, following the diet in its entirety 6 days a week, and including one "cheat" day a week when you include some foods which are not on the diet.

Again, understand that fitness has to be a lifetime commitment. Sit down and think what concrete changes you are willing to make – PERMANENTLY. Be specific. "I'll lose 5 pounds," is NOT good enough. Great, you lost five pounds. Now what? Same with, "I'll join a gym." You can join the gym but never go, or go, but spend your time socializing. What I mean by being specific, is something like, "I'll do 100 push-ups and 100 deep knee bends every day," or "I will eat at least 6 servings of fresh fruits and vegetables each day," or "I'll have one slice of cake on Saturday, but on no other days during the week." Once you have sat down and written your goals on paper, you are well on your way. Remember, you can always change your goals to suit your lifestyle. But it is important to have something objective on paper that you can follow.

Now that you have written down your plan, it's time to implement it. In order to be successful, think ahead and anticipate any problems that might arise. For example, how successful do you think you'll be at quitting smoking if you live with someone who smokes, or if you hang out in the bars every night with friends who smoke? How successful will you be at cutting down on junk food if every cabinet in your house is filled with cookies, chips and donuts, or if every day at work you get catered lunches?

One of the best ways to go about making lifestyle changes is to do it with your significant other. If you both decide to eat healthier, exercise, or quit smoking, it is easier than if just one of you does it. Enlisting the support of friends and family by sharing your goals with them can help as well. Make friendly bets about specific fitness goals.

Again, change specific things to implement your new lifestyle. Get rid of all of the junk food in your house. That way, even if you are tempted to indulge, you will have to go to the store to satisfy your cravings. Have plenty of healthy food available so that you have something to eat when hungry without having to go for the junk food.

Another suggestion is to take all of the money you spend buying junk from the vending machine each day, and put it aside. At the end of the month, take that money, and buy yourself something nice with it. Also, if part of your plan includes avoiding the fattening take-out or catered lunches at your office, make sure you bring a healthy lunch from home. If part of your job entails frequent business lunches, think about what you order, and watch those cocktails.

Many of you out there might be binge eaters. You will work out and follow a strict diet for a few months, only to mess things up when you start binging on your favorite food because of stress, lack of discipline, or a misguided notion that you'll only have one small piece of cake, or only binge this once. **If you find that you often ruin your diet by binging, it is important that you identify what foods you binge on and to avoid them at all cost.** For some of you it's chocolate, for others salty snacks such as chips and pretzels, and for some it's bread. Some are unfortunate and binge on many foods. Whatever your binge food or foods are, avoid them. Don't think you'll stop at just one serving.

If you are trying to quit smoking, make a specific plan. For example, you can decide to smoke one less cigarette a week until you quit. You can decide to only smoke after meals. Also, don't keep a pack on you – keep it in an inconvenient place such as the garage. This way, you'll have to actually get up from what you are doing to go for a smoke. Another suggestion is to do a set of push-ups, deep knee bends, jumping jacks, or some other exercise each time you want a cigarette. When you finish the exercise, decide if you still have the craving. You'll find that often times, performing the exercise will make you think about your health and you won't go smoke. Yet another suggestion is to keep a picture of your significant others and/or your children in your pack. Every time you want to smoke, think to yourself, "I might not live to see my daughter get married. I might not get to grow old with my husband. I might not live to see my son graduate from high school (yes, lung cancer can strike at a younger age too). I might not live to see my grandchildren." Then decide, is the cigarette still worth it?

Come up with your own ideas. There are endless possibilities. The point is to make a specific plan, anticipate any problems that might arise, make contingency plans for those problems, and then stick with it, refining your plan to suit your lifestyle.

There will be times when your program fails. For whatever reason, you relapse back to your old lifestyle. For example, we all know of people who at one point quit smoking but now smoke again, or someone who lost tons of weight but is now fatter than ever. The key is to get right back into it. **Reflect on the reason you failed.** It could be almost anything. **The plan might have been too strict or unrealistic.** For example, the average overweight, middle-aged man who hasn't exercised since high school will probably not be able to start with a regimen of 500 push-ups and 500 sit-ups every day. Similarly, for a person who is used to eating only processed junk food, switching to an all-natural diet cold turkey might be undoable, and a gradual changeover would be prudent. **Another reason for failure is a failure to come up with contingency plans for potential problems that might arise that derail you from your program. Look carefully and objectively at the circumstances that caused you to fail, and come up with specific ideas to fix the situation. Most importantly, don't beat yourself up if you went off of your diet or exercise regimen – it happens to the best of us. Just bounce back up and resume from where you left off.**

Eventually, you will find that your new fitness program becomes fully incorporated into your life to the point where the changes you have made become second nature. You will no longer be as tempted to cheat, and most likely, if you have stuck with an effective program, the positive changes in your body will help reinforce sticking to your program. HOWEVER – throughout your life, remain on guard. No matter how long you have stuck to your program, or how successful you have been, there is ALWAYS the possibility of relapse. For example, if you are starting college or a new stressful job, you might not be as careful about what you eat since it is not convenient, or you might find that you have less time to exercise. My advice is to adapt. Instead of scrapping your program, modify it to adapt to your new environment. For example, let's say you lost your job and thus don't have the money to go to a gym anymore. Instead of scrapping your program, adapt by working out at home using bodyweight exercises. If you suddenly find that a new job leaves you no time to exercise, use bodyweight exercises, and break up your routine so that you do perhaps 10 minutes when you wake up and 10 minutes before going to bed instead of a block of 20-30 minutes in the afternoon or evening when you don't have time. Be flexible.

Lastly, use the momentum you have gained from sticking to your program and seeing the positive changes in your body to incorporate more positive changes in your life. For example, if you have cut down on smoking, try to give it up completely. If you eliminated white flour and white sugar from your diet 6 days a week and lost some weight in the process, now maybe add a modest exercise program so that you can lose some more weight and build some muscle.

In conclusion, the way to successfully implement a fitness program is to: 1) Come up with a plan you know you can stick to for life, writing down every part of the plan specifically. 2) Anticipate any problems that might arise that would derail you from your goals and make contingency plans to counter those problems. 3) If you fail, look at why you failed, and think of ways to prevent failure in the future. 4) With time, your new fitness program will become easier and easier to follow, so build upon the positive changes your body has undergone, and include more positive changes.

Tamir B. Katz, M.D.

Part 4 – Advice for Healthy Living

Tamir B. Katz, M.D.

Stress

In life, our body is faced with two types of stress – acute and chronic. An acute stress is a specific occurrence that happens to your body which your body has to deal with. Being chased by someone, worrying about a final exam, suffering a heart attack, twisting your ankle, breaking your wrist, getting drunk, overeating, and staying up all night are all examples. The body can deal with an acute stress in one of two ways. It either gets through it, or else it breaks down, in which case you either suffer harm or death. For example, say you drank one too many shots of whiskey. Your body either succeeds in metabolizing the alcohol or vomiting it out, or else your body fails and you develop acute pancreatitis or alcohol poisoning, both of which may kill you. Another example is stressing over your final exam. The exam passes and your body emerges unscathed, or else the stress of worrying about it, coupled with the stress of staying up all night studying, weaken your immune system and you catch a cold. You should try to limit severe acute stresses in your life, such as drinking too much alcohol, or breaking a bone, but some stress is perfectly fine, and your body is well equipped to handle it.

A chronic stress is a series of acute stresses. For example, if you drink a bottle of vodka every day, or smoke every day, eat the wrong foods most of the time, have constant stress at work or home, or run 20 miles a day, your body is under chronic stress. The body was not designed to deal with chronic stresses. It does its best to adapt, but the result is a mal-adaption. For example, in someone who eats too much of the wrong foods every day, the body often "adapts" with obesity. When faced with chronic excessive alcohol consumption, the body attempts to adapt in other ways such as producing more enzymes to metabolize the alcohol. However, this in turn allows more alcohol to be consumed, leading to more damage. **The bottom line is that the end result of chronic stress is disease, since at some point the body cannot overcome the stress placed on it any more and it "breaks**

down." Thus, your goal should be to limit the amount of chronic stress that your body has to deal with. Let's go through the various aspects of life and see where we can reduce chronic stress.

We'll start with your job. Job stress is the cause of many illnesses both directly and indirectly. It directly damages your body by flooding it with catabolic stress hormones. The more you're stressed, the more stress hormones are released and flow through you, breaking down muscle and otherwise weakening your body. Of course stress hormones have their function in the body such as when you're in danger, sick, or injured. However, your body was not meant to deal with such high levels of stress hormones on a daily basis.

Indirectly, job stress causes damage because it is linked to smoking, drinking, drug abuse, and overeating junk foods, all of which are ways people use to cope with stress.

The bottom line is that you must start reducing job stress as much as you can. Many of you spend a significant chunk of your lives at work, and if the work environment is extremely stressful, it can take its toll on your health. Look inside as well. Are you the type of person that places work above all else? Maybe its time to start prioritizing. A job is important, but there is (or should be) more to life. When you're old, do you want to look back at your life as one long office day, or do you want to have fond memories of the quality times you enjoyed with family, friends, and loved ones, or of the times you helped people out through good deeds? I can't answer these questions for you. I just want you to stop and think before you overwork yourself to an early grave.

Job stress can also be related to exposure to harmful substances at work, including asbestos, coal dust, molds, carcinogenic chemicals, and radiation. Exposing yourselves to these substances day after day places an enormous chronic stress on your body's defense mechanisms, potentially leading to cancer. So protect yourselves, or if you have to, switch jobs. At the very least, educate yourself as to what kind of potential harmful substances you are being exposed to and what you can do to protect yourself.

Finally, on the way to work and back exists stress from traffic. How many of you get furious when someone cuts you off or drives too slowly? Believe me, it's not worth it. Let him cut you off. You'll arrive at your destination in the same amount of time without ruining your health or risking your life in the process. If you find that you really can't control your emotions when driving, seriously consider public transportation and/or carpooling.

Another source of stress is at home, stemming from financial, marital, or family-related problems. This is not the forum to discuss such problems, and I am by no means an expert, but I do suggest that you do try to do something about whatever problems you have. There are many qualified professionals out there who can help you. But it's up to you to take the first step and seek that help.

Yet another source of stress can come from our food. Even if you are following a healthy diet, many foods will have minute concentrations of toxins. Your body can readily deactivate these, but if you always consume the same foods, day in and day out, these toxins might at some point overwhelm your body's mechanisms for getting rid of them, potentially causing harm.

Thus, VARIETY IS ESSENTIAL. Try to eat different foods. Experiment. A major part of the problem with conventional diets is that they are built around very few types of food, namely a handful of grains, dairy products, and sweeteners. Hunter-gatherer diets such as the TBK Diet offer a huge variety of different foods. **You don't have to eat different things every day, but do make sure to vary your diet from time to time.**

Food can also be a cause of stress through gluttony. Although you should eat whenever hungry, do not pig out or stuff yourself. No matter how healthy a food is, chronic overeating strains the entire body.

Chronic stress from alcohol, tobacco, and drug abuse is an especially large problem in our society. Unfortunately, people often use these as ways to cope with stress on the job or at home. The result is a constant bombardment of caustic poison which ultimately destroys your body. Do all that you can to rid yourself of these harmful vices.

Although you cannot always reduce the amount of stress in your life, there are ways to deal with it in a healthier manner. Exercise is a great example. Prayer and spirituality are another great way. The following technique can help as well. Follow it for 5-20 or more minutes every day. Pick a word or phrase which brings to mind relaxation or peace. It could be anything, such as "All is well," "Everything is fine," or "All is peaceful." Sit or even lie down in a comfortable place. Close your eyes, completely relax your entire body from head to toe, and begin saying your phrase or word over and over again, in a soft voice or silently to yourself. At the same time, take long deep breaths, and block out all other thoughts from your mind besides the phrase or word. Initially, when you start out, thoughts will enter your mind against your control. When this happens, simply push them out without getting disturbed, and continue focusing solely on your phrase.

I want to emphasize that feeling stressed out is not "all in your head." You're not mentally ill if your body feels sick from stress. Actual destructive physiological changes occur in the body during periods of chronic stress. It is of the utmost importance that you not be bashful or feel too embarrassed to seek help if you need it. There are plenty of good therapists, psychologists, and psychiatrists out there, all of who can help you. However, it is up to you to do something about it. This is true of depression as well. Depression can take its toll on the body. Seek help. It is out there.

Hygiene

Hygiene is an important component of staying healthy, as well as preventing the spread of disease. Washing your hands, especially if you work with people, is an important way of preventing the spread of many illnesses. A large reason patients suffer complications while in the hospital is from lack of consistent hand washing on the part of health care practitioners. Many of the food poisoning outbreaks also occur from poor hygiene and not washing one's hand after using the bathroom (thus cooking your own food is the way to go).

Good dental hygiene through regular brushing, flossing, and dental cleanings is essential as well. Many types of bacteria thrive in your mouth, including one species that is known to damage the heart valves. Having sick gums that bleed make it easy for the bacteria to reach the bloodstream. By following a hunter-gatherer type diet such as the TBK Diet, free from starches and sugars, you are already decreasing your chances of developing cavities (dried fruit and fruit juice can cause cavities as well, so therefore it is best not to overindulge). If you smoke or abuse alcohol, it is especially important to take care of your teeth and visit the dentist, since these two vices cause a lot of damage to the mouth and gums.

Check-ups and Preventive Medicine

Getting a check up from your physician, especially if you are middle-aged or older, or have a strong family history of a particular disease at an early age, is a good idea. There are several screening tests available today which can often detect illness at an early stage and thus allow early intervention and a good prognosis. Checking your blood pressure and controlling it early on in life is important for prevention of the serious complications of high blood pressure such as stroke, heart disease, and kidney failure. A fasting cholesterol test, along with triglycerides, fasting glucose levels, and even homocysteine levels are worthwhile tests to do as you approach middle age or have a strong family history of heart disease or diabetes. However, be aware that a total cholesterol level of under 160 has been associated with increased mortality from non-cardiac causes such as cancer. So don't become obsessed with the numbers. Your HDL level is more important. Data from the long running Framingham Study has shown a U-shaped mortality curve. At cholesterols above 240, deaths from heart attacks skyrocketed, and below 160, deaths from other causes skyrocketed. So what's a healthy cholesterol to have? Well, a level of 165-200 or so is probably fine as long as your HDL level is high (at least 50) triglyceride levels are normal (100 or less), your fasting glucose is normal (ideally less than 100 as well), and you are of normal weight. Even if you do have high cholesterol levels, there is a very effective group of medications known as statins which lower your LDL levels while increasing HDL levels. Talk to your physician for more information.

Everyone over the age of 50 (younger if there is a family history) should get a colonoscopy. With such a marvelous technique at hand, there is no reason anyone should be developing colon cancer today. Opt for a colonoscopy instead of a sigmoidoscopy, which only covers the third of the colon where tumors are most likely to occur, but doesn't examine the rest of the colon. Mammograms are recommended for women for early detection of breast cancer. Women over the age of 40 might benefit from a mammogram every 2 years, and those over 50 for sure should go for one (again, if there is a family history of breast cancer, ask your physician about doing a mammogram even earlier). A PSA test for prostate cancer is also something to ask your physician about, but as of this writing, there haven't been any formal recommendations made. Pap smears have revolutionized early detection of cervical cancer to the extent that there is no reason that any woman has to develop that awful disease.

There are many other tests available, but it is important that you understand the following points. First off, all the screening tests in the world are no substitute for a healthy lifestyle. You will still get sick if you take poor care of yourself. The screening tests are mainly tools to give you a second chance to take charge of your health. Also, although going to the doctor and getting the various tests out there are important, overdoing it is not good either. For the average, healthy person, there is no need to constantly be checking everything out. Such obsessions can only lead to high levels of anxiety and stress.

Donating Blood

If you're a healthy man or a postmenopausal woman, **with your physician's permission,** donate blood 3-4 times a year or so. It turns out that our bodies often store too much iron, which is commonly found in many different foods, and in excess amounts may lead to heart disease and cancer. Storing iron is a natural adaptation, since in nature, humans coexist with parasites, which unload from us of some of our blood and the iron stored within. The problem is that nowadays, most of us are not infested with parasites, and so with the exception of menstruating women, many of us have high iron levels. You can check your iron levels with a simple blood test, so again, speak to your physician.

Hormone Replacement Therapy

Many women, upon reaching menopause, opt for hormone replacement therapy (HRT) to relieve hot flashes and to prevent osteoporosis and heart disease. **However, it has been recently discovered that women taking the most common form of HRT actually have an INCREASED risk of developing heart disease, as well as strokes, blood clots, and breast cancer.** If you are currently on HRT, I would strongly advise you to make an appointment with your physician to discuss discontinuing it. **However, don't stop abruptly by yourself, speak to your physician.** HRT has been shown to protect against colon cancer and osteoporosis, but in light of the fact that colonoscopies detect colonic polyps and tumors extremely well, and that a good diet along with weight bearing exercises can slow down or prevent osteoporosis, I fail to see a benefit in continuing HRT for most women.

Sunlight

Get some sunlight when you can. Don't overdo it, but don't run away from the sun either, and don't always opt for the sunscreen lotion. Sunscreen and protective clothes are for those times when you're going to be out in the sun for a while, or when the sun is at its hottest during midday. Ten or more minutes (depending on your skin type) of sunlight a day is healthy, supplying your body with vitamin D, which helps build strong bones and may protect against certain forms of cancer.

Massage

Whenever you have time, and especially after working out, massage your muscles by rubbing them, squeezing them, rolling and kneading them like you would dough, and by pressing down with your thumb into the muscle and moving it in small circular movements. Massage your feet, calves, thighs, lower back, abdomen, chest, arms, wrists, hands, shoulders, neck, and scalp. Have a loved one give you a massage, and reciprocate by giving him or her one as well. A good massage will relieve stress, help you recover from a strenuous workout, and generally provide you with a feeling of relaxation.

Tamir B. Katz, M.D.

Part 5 – Bibliography

Articles

Heart Disease & Stroke:

Albert C, et al. Blood Levels of Long Chain n-3 Fatty Acids and the Risk of Sudden Death. *New England Journal of Medicine.* 2002;346:1113-1118

Ascherio A, Willett WC. Health Effects of Trans Fatty Acids. *American Journal of Clinical Nutrition.* 1997;66:1006S-10S.

Ascherio A, et al. Dietary Fat and Risk of Coronary Heart Disease in Men: Cohort Follow Up Study in the United States. *BMJ.* 1996;313:84-90.

Bantle JP, et al. Effects of Dietary Fructose on Plasma Lipids in Healthy Subjects. *American Journal of Clinical Nutrition.* 2000;72:1128-34.

Bazzano LA, et al. Fruit and Vegetable Intake and Risk of Cardiovascular Disease in U.S. Adults: the First National Health and Nutrition Examination Survey Epidemiologic Follow-up Study. *American Journal of Clinical Nutrition.* 2002;76:93-9.

Beilin LJ. Vegetarian and Other Complex Diets, Fats, Fiber, and Hypertension. *American Journal of Clinical Nutrition.* 1994;59:1130S-5S.

Berglund L, et al. HDL – Subpopulation Patterns in Response to Reductions in Dietary Total and Saturated Fat Intakes in Healthy Subjects. *American Journal of Clinical Nutrition.* 1999;70:992-1000.

Brown BG, et al. Simvastatin and Niacin, Antioxidant Vitamins, or the Combination for the Prevention of Coronary Disease. *New England Journal of Medicine.* 2001;345:1583-92.

Dewailly E, et al. Cardivascular Disease Risk Factors and n-3 Fatty Acid Status in the Adult Population of James Bay Cree. *American Journal of Clinical Nutrition.* 2002;76:85-92.

Dewailly E, et al. n-3 Fatty Acids and Cardiovascular Disease Risk Factors Among the Inuit of Nunavik. *American Journal of Clinical Nutrition.* 2001;74:464-73.

Dreon DM, et al. A Very-Low-Fat Diet is Not Associated with Improved Lipoprotein Profiles in Men with a Predominance of Large, Low-Density Lipoproteins. *American Journal of Clinical Nutrition.* 1999;69:411-8.

Dreon DM, et al. Change in Dietary Saturated Fat Intake is Correlated With Change in Mass of Large Low-Density-Lipoprotein Particles in Men. *American Journal of Clinical Nutrition.* 1998;67:828-36.

Feldman EB. Assorted Monounsaturated Fatty Acids Promote Healthy Hearts. *American Journal of Clinical Nutrition.* 1999;70:953-4.

Felton CV, et al. Dietary Polyunsaturated Fatty Acids and Composition of Arterial Plaques. *Lancet.* 1994;322:1195-6.

Gaziano JM, Manson JE. Changing the Natural History of Coronary Heart Disease. *Cardiology Clinics.* 1996;14:69-83.

Gillman MW, et al. Inverse Association of Dietary Fat with Development of Ischemic Stroke in Men. *JAMA.* 1997;278:2145-50.

Golomb BA. Dietary Fats and Heart Disease – Dogma Challenged? *Journal of Clinical Epidemiology.* 1998;51:461-4.

Grant WB. Milk and Other Dietary Influences on Coronary Heart Disease. *Alternative Medicine Review.* 1998;3:281-94.

Havel RJ. Genetic Underpinnings of LDL Size and Density: a Role for Hepatic Lipase? *American Journal of Clinical Nutrition.* 2000;71:1390-1.

Hu FB, et al. Dietary Protein and Risk of Ischemic Heart Disease in Women. *American Journal of Clinical Nutrition.* 1999;70:221-7.

Hu FB, et al. Dietary Fat Intake and the Risk of Coronary Heart Disease in Women. *New England Journal of Medicine.* 1997;337:1491-9.

Jee SA, et al. Coffee Consumption and Serum Lipids: A Meta-Analysis of Randomized Controlled Clinical Trials. *American Journal of Epidemiology.* 2001;153:353-62.

Kamigaki AS, et al. Low Density Lipoprotein Partical Size and Risk of Early-Onset Myocardial Infarction in Women. *American Journal of Epidemiology.* 2001;153:939-945.

Kasim-Karakas SE, et al. Changes in Plasma Lipoproteins During Low-Fat, High-Carbohydrate Diets: Effects of Energy Intake. *American Journal of Clinical Nutrition.* 2000:1439-47.

Katan MB. Effect of Low-Fat Diets on Plasma High-Density Lipoprotein Concentraitions. *American Journal of Clinical Nutrition.* 1998;67:573S-6S.

Katan MB, Grundy SM, Willett WC. Beyond Low-Fat Diets. *New England Journal of Medicine.* 1997;337:563-6.

Kritchevsky D. Diet and Atherosclerosis. *American Heart Journal.* 1999;138:426S-30S.

Kummerow FA, Zhou Q, Mahfouz MM. Effect of Trans Fatty Acids on Calcium Influx into Human Arterial Endothelial Cells. *American Journal of Clinical Nutrition.* 1999;70:832-8.

Lamaroche B, et al. Fasting Insulin and Apolipoprotein B Levels and Low-Density Lipoprotein Particle Size as Risk Factors for Ischemic Heart Disease. *JAMA.* 1998;279:1955-61.

Lauer MS. Aspirin for Primary Prevention of Coronary Events. *New England Journal of Medicine.* 2002;346:1468-74.

Leeds AR. Glycemic Index and Heart Disease. *American Journal of Clinical Nutrition.* 2002;76:286S-9S

Lewis NM, Schalch K, Scheideler SE. Serum Lipid Response to n-3 Fatty Acid Enriched Eggs in Persons With Hypercholesterolemia. *Journal of the American Dietetic Association.* 2000;100:365-7.

Lindeberg S, et al. Age Relations of Cardiovascular Risk Factors in a Traditional Melanesian Society: the Kitava Study. *American Journal of Clinical Nutrition.* 1997;66:845-52.

Lindeberg S, et al. Haemostatic Variables in Pacific Islanders apparently Free From Stroke and Ischaemic Heart Disease – The Kitava Study. *Thrombosis and Haemostasis.* 1997;77:94-8.

Lindeberg S, et al. Cardivascular Risk Factors in a Melanesian Population Apparently Free from Stroke and Ischaemic Heart Disease: the Kitava Study. *Journal of Internal Medicine.* 1994;236:331-40.

Lindeberg S, Lundh B. Apparent Absence of Stroke and Ischaemic Heart Disease in a Traditional Melanesian Island: a Clinical Study in Kitava. *Journal of Internal Medicine.* 1993;233:269-75.

Liu S, et al. Relation Between a Diet with a High Glycemic Load and Plasma Concentrations of High Sensitivity C-reactive Protein in Middle-Aged Women. *American Journal of Clinical Nutrition.* 2002;75:492-8.

Liu S, et al. Dietary Glycemic Load Assessed by Food-Frequency Questionnaire in Relation to Plasma High-Density-Lipoprotein Cholesterol and Fasting Plasma Triacylglycerols in Postmenopausal Women. *American Journal of Clinical Nutrition.* 2001;73:560-6.

Liu S, et al. A prospective Study of Dietary Glycemic Load, Carbohydrate Intake, and Risk of Coronary Heart Disease in US Women. *American Journal of Clinical Nutrition.* 2000;71:1455-61.

Louheranta AM, et al. Linoleic Acid Intake and Susceptibility of Very-Low and Low-Density Lipoproteins to Oxidation in Men. *American Journal of Clinical Nutrition.* 1996;63:698-703.

Meagher EA, et al. Effects of Vitamin E on Lipid Peroxidation in Healthy Persons. *JAMA.* 2001;285:1178-82.

Morgan WA, Clayshulte BJ. Pecans Lower Low-Density Lipoprotein Cholesterol in People with Normal Lipid Levels. *Journal of the American Dietetic Association.* 2000;100:312-18.

Multiple Risk Factor Intervention Trial Research Group. Multiple Risk Factor Intervention Trial. *JAMA.* 1982;248:1465-77.

Oliver MF. It Is More Important to Increase the Intake of Unsaturated Fats Than to Decrease the Intake of Saturated Fats: Evidence From Clinical Trials Relating To Ischemic Heart Disease. *American Journal of Clinical Nutrition.* 1997;66:980S-6S.

Oomen CM, et al. Fish Consumption and Coronary Heart Disease Mortality in Finland, Italy, and the Netherlands. *American Journal of Epidemiology.* 2000;151:999-1006.

Pietinen P, et al. Intake of Fatty Acids and Risk of Coronary Heart Disease in a Cohort of Finnish Men: The Alpha-Tocopherol, Beta-Carotene Cancer Prevention Study. *American Journal of Epidemiology.* 1997;145:876-87.

Prior IA, et al. Cholesterol, Coconuts, and Diet on Polynesian Atolls: a Natural Experiment: the Pukapuka and Tokelau Island Studies. *American Journal of Clinical Nutrition.* 1981;34:1552-61.

Raeini-Sarjaz M, et al. Comparison of the Effect of Dietary Fat Restriction With That of Energy Restriction on Human Human Lipid Metabolism. *American Journal of Clinical Nutrition.* 2001;73:262-7.

Ravnskov U. The Questionable Role of Saturated and Polyunsaturated Fatty Acids in Cardiovascular Disease. *Journal of Clinical Epidemiology.* 1998;51:443-60.

Renaud S, De Lorgeril M. Wine, Alcohol, Platelets, and the French Paradox for Coronary Heart Disease. *Lancet.* 1992;339:1523-6.

Rimm EB, et al. Folate and Vitamin B6 From Diet and Supplements in Relation to Risk of Coronary Heart Disease Among Women. *JAMA.* 1998;279:359-64.

Rosenberg IH. Fish-Food to Calm the Heart. *New England Journal of Medicine.* 2001;346:1102-3.

Sabate` J. Nut Consumption, Vegetarian Diets, Ischemic Heart Disease Risk, and All-Cause Mortality: Evidence From Epidemiologic Studies. *American Journal of Clinical Nutrition.* 1999;70:500S-3S.

Schaefer EJ, Brousseau ME. Diet, Lipoproteins, and Coronary Heart Disease. *Endocrinology and Metabolism Clinics.* 1998;27:712-32.

Schyder Guido, et al. Decreased Rate of Coronary Restenosis After Lowering of Plasma Homocysteine Levels. *New England Journal of Medicine.* 2001;345:1593-1600.

Serra-Majem L, et al. How Could Changes in Diet Explain Changes in Coronary Heart Disease Mortality in Spain? The Spanish Paradox. *American Journal of Clinical Nutrition.* 1995;61:1351S-9S.

Shaper AG. Cardiovascular Studies in the Samburu Tribe of Northern Kenya. *American Heart Journal.* 1962;63:437-42.

Taubes G. The Soft Science of Dietary Fat. *Science.* 2001;291:2536-2545.

Toborek M, et al. Unsaturated Fatty Acids Selectively Induce an Inflammatory Environment in Human Endothelial Cells. *American Journal of Clinical Nutrition. 2002;75:119-25.*

Ulbricht TLV, Southgate DAT. Coronary Heart Disease: Seven Dietary Factors. *Lancet.* 1991;338:985-92.

Urgert R, et al. Separate Effects of the Coffee Diterpenes Cafesol and Kahweol on Serum Lipids and Liver Aminotransferases. *American Journal of Clinical Nutrition.* 1997;65:519-24.

Vasan RS. *New England Journal of Medicine.* 2002;347:305-313, 358-9.

Williams PT, Krauss RM. Low-Fat Diets, Lipoprotein Subclasses, and Heart Disease Risk. *American Journal of Clinical Nutrition.* 1999;70:949-50.

Yu JN, et al. Hyperlipidemia. Primary Care; Clinics in Office Practice. 2000;27.

Diabetes:

Berry EM. Dietary Fatty Acids in the Management of Diabetes Mellitus. *American Journal of Clinical Nutrition.* 1997;66:991S-7S.

Brand Miller JC, Colagiuri S. The Carnivore Connection: Dietary Carbohydrate in the Evolution of NIDDM. *Diabetologia.* 1994;37:1280-6.

Buyken AE, et al. Glycemic Index in the Diet of European Outpatients with Type 1 Diabetes: Relations to Glycated Hemoglobin and Serum Lipids. *American Journal of Clinical Nutrition.* 2001;73:574-81.

Garg A, et al. Effects of varying Carbohydrate Content of Diet in Patients With Non-Insulin-Dependent Diabetes Mellitus. *JAMA.* 1994;271:1421-8.

Gerstein HC. Cow's Milk Exposure and Type-1 Diabetes Mellitus. *Diabetes Care.* 1994;17:13-19.

McDonald RB. Influence of Dietary Sucrose on Biological Aging. *American Journal of Clinical Nutrition.* 1995;62:284S-93S.

O'Dea K, et al. Impaired Glucose Tolerance, Hyperinsulinemia, and Hypertryglyceridemia in Australian Aborigines From the Desert. *Diabetes Care.* 1988;11:23-29.

Roslova H, Mayer Jr O, Reaven G. Effect of Variations in Plasma Magnesium Concentration on Resistence to Insulin Mediated Glucose Disposal in Nondiabetic Subjects. *Journal of Clinical Endocrinology and Metabolism.* 1997;82:3783-5.

Salmeron J, et al. Dietary Fat Intake and Risk of Type 2 Diabetes in Women. *American Journal of Clinical Nutrition.* 2001;73:1019-26.

Saukkonen T, et al. Significance of Cow's Milk Protein Antibodies as Risk Factor for Childhood IDDM: Interactions with Dietary Cow's Milk Intake and HLA-DQB1 Genotype. *Diabetologia.* 1998;41:72-8.

Scott FW, Norris JM, Kolb H. Milk and Type-1 Diabetes: Examining the Evidence and Broadening the Focus. *Diabetes Care.* 1996;19:379-83.

Walker KZ, et al. Body Fat Distribution and Non-Insulin-Dependent Diabetes: Comparison of a Fiber-Rich, High Carbohydrate, Low-Fat (23%) Diet and a 35% Fat Diet High in Monounsaturated Fat. *American Journal of Clinical Nutrition.* 1996;63:254-60.

Willet W, Manson J, Liu S. Glycemic Index, Glycemic Load, and Risk of Type 2 Diabetes. *American Journal of Clinical Nutrition.* 2002;76:274S-80S.

Cancer:

Augustsson K, et al. Dietary Heterocyclic Amines and Cancer of the Colon, Rectum, Bladder, and Kidney: a Population Based Study. *Lancet.* 1999;353:703-7.

Bingham SA. High-Meat Diets and Cancer Risk. *Proceedings of the Nutrition Society.* 1999;58:243-8.

Bostick RM, et al. Sugar, Meat, and Fat Intake, and Non-Dietary Risk Factors for Colon Cancer Incidence in Iowa Women (United States). *Cancer Causes & Control.* 1994;5:38-52.

Bruce WR, Wolever TMS, Giacca A. Mechanisms Linking Diet and Colorectal Cancer: The Possible Role of Insulin Resistance. *Nutrition and Cancer.* 2000;37:19-26.

Chan JM, et al. Dairy Products, Calcium, and Prostate Cancer Risk in the Physicians Health Study. *American Journal of Clinical Nutrition.* 2001;74:549-54.

Chatenoud L, et al. Refined Cereal Intake and Risk of Selected Cancers in Italy. *American Journal of Clinical Nutrition.* 1999;70:1107-10.

Davies TW, et al. Adolescent Milk, Dairy Product and Fruit Consumption and Testicular Cancer. *British Medical Journal.* 1996;74:657-60.

Fernandez E, et al. Fish Consumption and Cancer Risk. *American Journal of Clinical Nutrition.* 1999;70:85-90.

Forman D. Meat and Cancer: a Relation in Search of a Mechanism. *Lancet.* 1999;353:686-7.

Franceschi S, et al. Intake of Macronutrients and Risk of Breast Cancer. *Lancet.* 1996;347:1351-6.

Frentzel-Beyme R, Chang-Claude J. Vegetarian Diets and Colon Cancer: the German Experience. *American Journal of Clinical Nutrition.* 1994;59:1143S-52S.

Giovannucci E, et al. Intake of Fat, Meat, and Fiber in Relation to Risk of Colon Cancer in Men. *Journal of Cancer Research.* 1994;54:2390-7.

Goldbohm RA, et al. A Prospective Cohort Study on the Relation Between Meat Consumption and the Risk of Colon Cancer. *Journal of Cancer Research.* 1994;54:718-23.

Hensrud DD, Heimburger DC. Nutritional Physiologic, and Pathophysiologic Considerations of the Gastrointestinal Tract. *Gastroenterology Clinics.* 1998;27:325-46.

Holmes MD, et al. Association of Dietary Intake of Fat and Fatty Acids With Risk of Breast Cancer. *JAMA.* 1999;281:914-920.

Hu J, et al. Diet and Cancer of the Stomach: A Case Control Study in China. *International Journal of Cancer.* 1988;41:331-5.

Kampman E, et al. Meat Consumption, Genetic Susceptibility, and Colon Cancer Risk: a United States Multicenter Case-Control Study. *Cancer Epidemiology, Biomarkers & Prevention.* 1999;8:15-24.

Kampman E, et al. Vegetable and Animal Products as Determinants of Colon Cancer Risk in Dutch Men and Women. *Cancer Causes & Control.* 1995;6:225-34.

Kaplan S, Novikov I, Modan B. Nutritional Factors in the Etiology or Brain Factors: Potential Role of Nitrosamines, Fat, and Cholesterol. *American Journal of Epidemiology.* 1997;146:832-41.

Kroser JA, Bachwich DR, Lichtenstein GR. Colorectal CarcinomaL Risk Factors for the Development of Colorectal Carcinoma and Their Modification. *Hemotolgy/Oncology Clinics of North America.* 1997;11:547-77.

La Vecchia C, et al. A Case-Control Study of Diet and Colo-Rectal Cancer in Northern Italy. *International Journal of Cancer.* 1988;41:492-8.

Michaud DS. A Prospective Study on Intake of Animal Products and Risk of Prostate Cancer. *Cancer Causes Control.* 2001;12(6):557-67.

Mills PK, et al. Cancer Incidence Among California Seventh-Day Adventists, 1976-1982. *American Journal of Clinical Nutrition.* 1994;59:1136S-42S.

Missmer SA. Meat and Dairy Food Consumption and Breast Cancer: a Pooled Analysis of Cohort Studies. *International Journal of Epidemiology.* 2002;31:78-85

Murphy TK, et al. Body Mass Index and Colon Cancer Mortality in a Large Prospective Study. *American Journal of Epidemiology.* 2000;152:847-54.

Rose DP. Dietary Fatty Acids and Cancer. *American Journal of Clinical Nutrition.* 1997;66:998S-1003S.

Rose DP and Connolly JM. Regulation of Tumor Angiogenesis by Dietary Fatty Acids and Eicosanoids. *Nutrition and Cancer.* 2000;37:119-27.

Slattery ML, et al. Dietary Energy Sources and Colon Cancer Risk. *American Journal of Epidemiology.* 1997;145:199-210.

Steinmaus CM, Nunez S, Smith AH. Diet and Bladder Cancer: A Meta-Analysis of Six Dietary Variables. *American Journal of Epidemiology.* 2000;151:693-702.

Steinmetz KA, Potter JD. Food-Group Consumption and Colon Cancer in the Adelaide Case-Control Study II. Meat, Poultry, Seafood, Dairy Foods, and Eggs. *International Journal of Cancer.* 1993;53:720-7.

Thun MT, et al. Risk Factors for Fatal Colon Cancer in a Large Prospective Study. *Journal of the National Cancer Institute.* 1992;82:1491-1500.

Voorhips LE, et al. Vegetable and Fruit Consumption and Risks of Colon and Rectal Cancer in a Prospective Cohort Study: The Netherlands Cohort Study on Diet and Cancer. *American Journal of Epidemiology.* 2000;152:1081-92.

Obesity:

Brand-Miller JC, et al. Glycemic Index and Obesity. *American Journal of Clinical Nutrition.* 2002;76:281S-5S.

Dennison BA, Rockwell HL, Baker SL. Excess Fruit Juice Consumption by Preschool-aged Children Is Associated With Short Stature and Obesity. *American Academy of Pediatrics.*1997;99:15-22.

Dorn JM, et al. Body Mass Index and Mortality in a General Population Sample of Men and Women: The Buffalo Health Study. *American Journal of Epidemiology.* 1997;146:919-31.

Rolls BJ, et al. Energy Density Not Fat Content of Foods Affected Energy Intake in Lean and Obese Women. *American Journal of Clinical Nutrition.* 1999;69:863-71.

Visscher TLS, et al. Underweight and Overweight in Relation to Mortality Among Men Aged 40-59 and 50-69 Years: The Seven Countries Study. *The American Journal of Epidemiology.* 2000;151:660-6.

Willet WC. Is Dietary Fat a Major Determinant of Body Fat? *American Journal of Clinical Nutrition.* 1998;67:556S-62S.

Willet WC. Dietary Fat and Obesity: an Unconvincing Relation. *American Journal of Clinical Nutrition.* 1998;68:1149-50.

Osteoporosis:

Hannan MT, et al. Effect of Dietary Protein on Bone Loss in Elderly Men and Women: The Framingham Osteoporosis Study. *American Society for Bone and Mineral Research.* 2000;15:2504-12.

Heaney RP. Protein Intake and Bone Health: the Influence of Belief Systems on the Conduct of Nutritional Source. *American Journal of Clinical Nutrition.* 2001;73:5-6.

Heaney RP. Dietary Protein and Phosphorous Do Not Affect Calcium Absorption. *American Journal of Clinical Nutrition.* 2000;72:758-61.

Munger RG, Cerhan JR, Chiu BCH. Prospective Study of Dietary Protein Intake and Risk of Hip Fracture in Postmenopausal Women. *American Journal of Clinical Nutrition.* 1999;69:147-52.

New SA, et al. Dietary Influences on Bone Mass and Bone Metabolism: Further Evidence of a Positive Link Between Fruit and Vegetable Consumption and Bone Health? *American Journal of Clinical Nutrition.* 2000;71:142-51.

Pannemans DLE, et al. Effect of Protein Source and Quantity on Protein Metabolism in Elderly Women. *American Journal of Clinical Nutrition.* 1998;68:1228-35.

Promislow JHE, et al. Protein Consumption and Bone Mineral Density in the Elderly. *American Journal of Epidemiology.* 2002;155:636-44.

Spencer, et al. Further Studies of the Effect of a High Protein Diet as Meat on Calcium Metabolism. *The American Journal of Clinical Nutrition.* 1983;37:924-9.

Tucker KL, et al. Potassium, Magnesium, and Fruit and Vegetable Intakes Are Associated with Greater Bone Mineral Density in Elderly Men and Women. *American Journal of Clinical Nutrition.* 1999;69:727-36.

Weinsier RL, Krumdieck CL. Dairy Foods and Bone Health: Examination of the Evidence. *American Journal of Clinical Nutrition.* 2000;72:681-9.

Wolf RL, et al. Factors Associated With Calcium Absorption Efficiency in Pre- and Perimenopausal Women. *American Journal of Clinical Nutrition.* 2000;72:466-71.

Miscellaneous:

Aldoori WH, et al. Prospective Study of Diet and the Risk of Duodenal Ulcer in Men. *American Journal of Epidemiology.* 1997;145:42-50.

Cordain L, et al. Plant-Animal Subsistence Ratios and Macronutrient Energy Estimates in Worldwide Hunter-Gatherer Diets. *American Journal of Clinical Nutrition.* 2000;71:682-92.

Eaton SB, Konner M. Paleolithic Nutrition: A Consideration of Its Nature and Current Implication. *New England Journal of Medicine.* 1985;312:283-9.

Fried LP, et al. Risk Factors for 5-Year Mortality in Older Adults. The Cardiovascular Health Study. *JAMA.* 1998;279:585-92.

Guthrie JF, Morton JF. Food Sources of Added Sweeteners in the Diets of Americans. *Journal of the American Dietetic Association.* 2000;100:43-48,51.

Foster-Powell K, Holt SHA, Brand-Miller JC. International Table of Glycemic Index and Glycemic Load Values: 2002. *American Journal of Clinical Nutrition.* 2002;76:5-56.

Haby MM, et al. Asthma in Preschool Children: Prevalence and Risk Factors. *Thorax.* 2001;56:589-95.

Jacobs DR, Iribarren C. Invited Commentary: Low Cholesterol and Nonatherosclerotic Disease Risk: A Persistently Perplexing Question. *American Journal of Epidemiology.* 2000;151:748-51.

Jenkins DJA, et al. Glycemic Index: Overview of Implications in Health and Disease. *American Journal of Clinical Nutrition.* 2002;76:266S-73S.

Key TJ, et al. Mortality in Vegetarians and Nonvegetarians: Detailed Findings from a Collaborative Analysis of 5 Perspective Studies. *American Journal of Clinical Nutrition.* 1999;70:516S-24S.

Larsson CL, Johansson GK. Dietary Intake and Nutritional Status of Young Vegans and Omnivores in Sweden. *American Journal of Clinical Nutrition.* 2002;76:100-6.

Lee M, Paffenbarger RS. Associations of Light, Moderate, and Vigorous Intensity Physical Activity with Longevity: The Harvard Alumni Health Study. *American Journal of Epidemiology.* 2000;151:293-9.

Linos A, et al. Dietary Factors in Relation to Rheumatoid Arthritis: a Role for Olive Oil and Cooked Vegetables? *American Journal of Clinical Nutrition.*1999;70:1077-82.

Ludwig DS, Eckel RH. The Glycemic Index at 20y. *American Journal of Clinical Nutrition.* 2002;76:264S-5S.

McCullough ML, et al. Adherence to the Dietary Guidelines for Americans and Risk of Major Chronic Disease in Women. *American Journal of Clinical Nutrition.* 2000;72:1214-22.

McCullough ML, et al. Adherence to the Dietary Guidelines for Americans and Risk of Major Chronic Disease in Men. *American Journal of Clinical Nutrition.* 2000;72:1223-31.

Molleson T. The Eloquent Bones of Abu Hureyra. *Scientific American.* August1994;70-5.

Nicklas TA, et al. Trends in Nutrient Intake of 10-Year-Old Children Over Two Decades (1973-1994): The Bogalusa Heart Study. *American Journal of Epidemiology.* 2001;153:969-77.

Rennie J. The Body Against Itself. *Scientific American.* December 1990;106-15.

Scrimshaw NS. Iron Deficiency. *Scientific American.* October 1991;46-52.

Song YM, Sung J, Kim JS. Which Cholesterol Level is Related to the Lowest Mortality in a Population with Mean Cholesterol Level: A 6.4-Year Follow-up Study of 482,472 Korean Men. *American Journal of Epidemiology.* 2000;151:739-47.

Von Boehmer H, Kisielow P. How the Immune System Learns About Self. *Scientific American.* October 1991;74-81.

Wurtman RJ, Wurtman JJ. Carbohydrates and Depression. *Scientific American.* January 1989:68-75.

Zhang SM, et al. Dietary Fat in Relation to Risk of Multiple Sclerosis Among Two Large Cohorts of Women. *American Journal of Epidemiology.* 2000;152:1056-64.

Books

Audette R. *Neanderthin.* St. Martin's Paperbacks. New York.1999.

Benson H. *The Relaxation Response.* Harpertorch. New York. 2000.

Bricklin M. Prevention Magazine's Nutrition Advisor. MJF Books. New York. 1993.

Cordain L. *The Paleodiet.* John Wiley & Sons, Inc. New York. 2002.

Eades MR, Eades MD. *The Protein Power Lifeplan.* Warner Books. New York. 2000.

Fauci AS, Braunwald E, Isselbacher KJ, Wilson JD, Martin JB, Kasper DL, Hauser SL, Longo DL, eds. *Harrison's Principles of Internal Medicine 14th Edition.* McGraw-Hill. 1998.

Griffin JE, Ojeda SR, eds. *Textbook of Endocrine Physiology 3rd Edition.* Oxford University Press. New York, Oxford. 1996;349-373.

Mount JL. *The Food and Health of Modern Man.* Charles Knight & Company Ltd. London & Tonbridge. 1975; 1-56,163-264.

Seely S, DLJ Freed, Sliverstone GA, Rippere V, eds. *Diet-Related Diseases: The Modern Epidemic.* Westport. AVI Publishing Co. 1985.

Shils ME, Olson JA, Shike M, eds. *Modern Nutrition in Health and Disease.* Lea & Febiger. Malvern, PA. 1993.

Zhuo D, Lade AR, Wong J. *Chinese Exercises & Massage For Health & Longevity.* Hartley & Marks Publishers. USA. 1998.

Tamir B. Katz, M.D.

For more information, please visit:
www.tbkfitness.org
or email:
tamirkatz@yahoo.com

About the Author

Tamir Katz is a graduate of SUNY Stony Brook School of Medicine and received a Bachelor's degree in Biology from Cornell University. He has been exploring different diets and exercise programs since 1993, and currently provides fitness and nutrition information through his website www.tbkfitness.org. Tamir lives in New York with his wife and daughter.

Printed in the United States
49402LVS00003B/157